PRAISE FOR JENNIFER ISERLOH

"*The Superfood Alchemy Cookbook* can help you get more creative in the kitchen and bring more intention and meaning into your daily routine. Jennifer Iserloh's plant-based recipes are nourishing, delicious, and super simple to make."

—AMANDA TUST, SENIOR EDITOR, *YOGA JOURNAL*

———◇———

"The foods you choose to eat can be the path to either pain or incredible healing. Learning to choose the right healing foods is the gift of *Superfood Alchemy*. Healing foods, especially 'good for your gut' superfoods, are the best medicine for a healthy life. Iserloh's book takes ancient wisdom that modern medicine is now beginning to embrace and powerfully delivers it in bite-sized chapters for our modern life. As a gut specialist, I say, keep this book in your kitchen to guide you on the best food choices for your total body wellness."

—VINCENT PEDRE, MD, BESTSELLING AUTHOR OF
*HAPPY GUT: THE CLEANSING PROGRAM TO HELP YOU
LOSE WEIGHT, GAIN ENERGY, AND ELIMINATE PAIN*

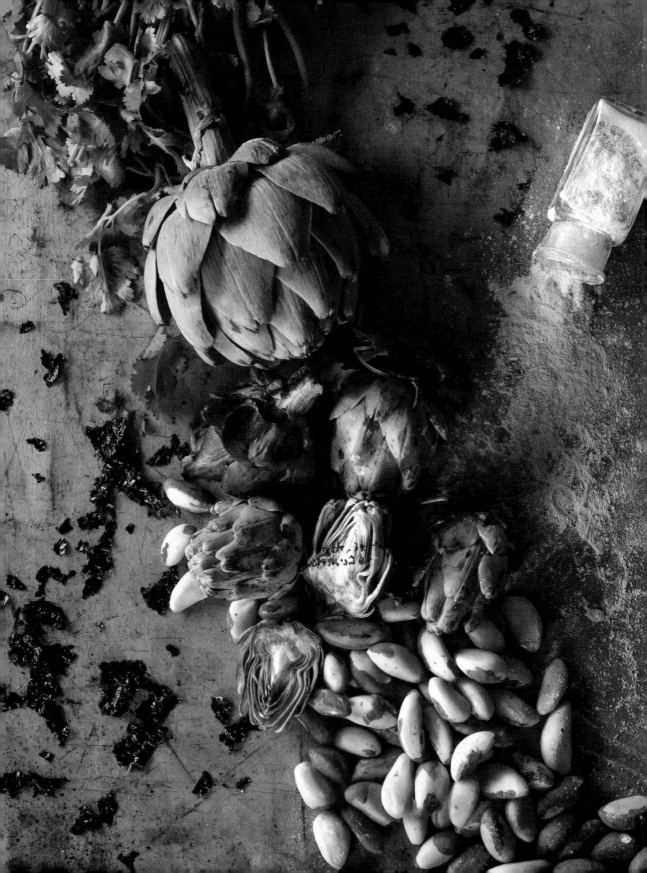

TRANSFORM *Nature's Most Powerful Ingredients into Nourishing Meals and Healing Remedies*

THE
Superfood Alchemy
COOKBOOK

JENNIFER ISERLOH

Da Capo
∞
LIFE
LONG

Da Capo Press
Hachette Book Group
1290 Avenue of the Americas,
New York, NY 10104
dacapopress.com
@DaCapoPress

Printed in the United States of America

First Edition: April 2019

Published by Da Capo Press, an imprint of Perseus Books, LLC, a subsidiary of Hachette Book Group, Inc.
The Da Capo Press name and logo is a trademark of the Hachette Book Group.

The publisher is not responsible for websites (or their content) that are not owned by the publisher.

Print book interior design by Tara Long/Dotted Line Design, llc.

Library of Congress Cataloging-in-Publication Data has been applied for.

ISBNs: 978-0-7382-8474-3 (paperback), 978-0-7382-8475-0 (ebook)

10 9 8 7 6 5 4 3 2 1

Contents

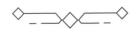

FOREWORD

by Sachin Patel, DC

When looking for the keys to better health, many of us head to the doctor's office in search of a magic fix. But health is so much more than just optimizing biochemistry and physiology. It's the balancing of body, mind, and spirit that creates true holistic health.

I work in the field of functional medicine, a progressive approach to health that looks at lifestyle as the key to healing. Food plays a huge role, along with emotional, environmental, and psychological factors. Before I found functional medicine, I thought I had my dream job in a busy practice working with world-class athletes. One day, a local TV station interviewed me about a case of severe pain that we were able to alleviate in a short time. Soon, our office was flooded with people who had many different types of chronic illnesses and complaints. I thought about referring these patients out, but many told me they had already been to other specialists, and the conventional medicine route had left them with no results. To address their issues, we had to look deeper.

This is when I discovered functional medicine. It looks at the root cause of illness, rather than just the symptoms. This resonated deeply with me. I immediately enrolled in a training program. During that time, I started to apply the principles on myself, realizing I had to clean up some of my own health practices. I had considered my own health issues to be "normal," since I thought my state was "just the way it is." Following the functional medicine route helped me to improve my health greatly by including foods, herbs, and mindfulness practices.

Traditional medicine views the body as hardware that can't be changed. In that view, DNA and genes are just part of your makeup, disease is an unavoidable part of your future based on the cards you were dealt, and food is just fuel to provide you with basic energy. In my view, food is the "software" that can override how your hardware works. This can create *very* different outcomes if you are using the right high-quality software, mainly functional foods—plant ingredients, superfoods, and healing herbs such as the ones in these recipes. Now, as the founder of the Living Proof Institute, serving hundreds of patients a year, I always turn to food, plants, and herbs for answers. We pair the right health-balancing foods with practices that support emotional health, the patient's goals, and purity of environment.

I practice one of the core principles of alchemy—the synergy between body, mind, and spirit—in a modern way. The effect of emotional health and mind-set on the body has long been ignored in Western medicine. These areas play a big role in how healthy and happy you are, and even how you make your food choices. One of my mantras is "Feel better, heal better." This is true not only for the emotional quality of your life, but also for biological reasons. By triggering stress hormones and blocking relaxation cues, low moods, stress, anger, and fear can offset how well your nervous system and gut work. The body heals best when it's in a state of parasympathetic balance. Being emotionally balanced with low stress levels means you're in that mode more often.

I have seen the power of synergies and connection in healing my patients' body, soul, and mind. I believe we can use cosmic intelligence—healing foods, seasonal eating, and getting out in nature, paired with testing, clinical goals, and improving mind-set—to reach a state of health we all long for, whether we're dealing with particular health concerns or looking to reach a higher level. With awesome plant-based dishes and meditation practices, *The Superfood Alchemy Cookbook* is the perfect how-to manual.

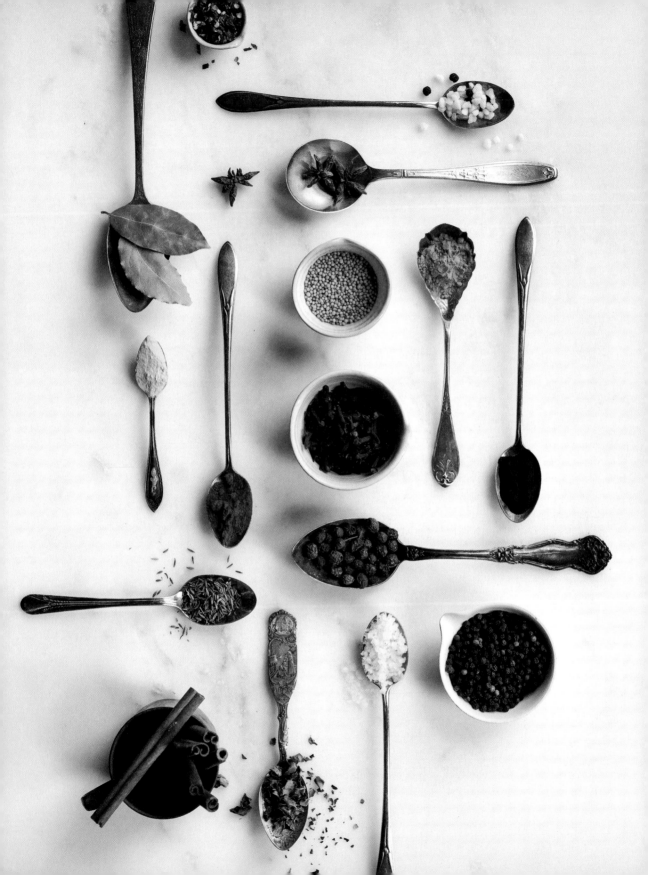

INTRODUCTION

As a veteran health writer/self-help junkie, chef, and yoga teacher, I have seen it all when it comes to health programs: countless books, diets, and gurus promising everything from weight loss to earning more money and increasing self-esteem. Before I started working with alchemy, I was trying to juggle my mind/body/soul practices separately, following some of these programs, and driving myself a bit crazy in the process—not finding quite what I was looking for and feeling like a hamster in the wheel of life. Eventually I went through a health "plateau" where even my yoga and meditation practice became stagnant and worn out. To an outside observer, I was living a dream life: I had a loving marriage, a stable income, and a fulfilling career. Yet I still felt something was missing. I felt that I still "hadn't made it" and was constantly feeling overwhelmed and frazzled, not a very healthy place to be mentally and emotionally. At the time, I chalked it up to being in my forties. Plus, I had to acknowledge that my career was exhaustingly action-packed—years of working long, intense hours in the New York City fine dining scene; leaving the restaurant business to become a writer and penning more than twenty books; and continuing my education from yoga teacher to certified holistic-health coach, Reiki healer, and more. No wonder I was tired, right?

I was very discouraged and beginning to feel stuck, but still maintained an intense love of food and cooking. I knew there must be something out there that could help me break through to the next level. Then one day, I saw an old alchemy drawing, an obscure engraving from the 1700s called the *Tabula Smaragdina* (which translates to "Emerald Tablet"). It's a pictorial representation of the alchemy formula that teaches you the path to "deepest transformation," how to become more evolved in mind, body, and soul—in other words, to achieve a more healthy, vibrant, enriching life. Alchemy teaches us that healthy living practices must be universally integrated to be truly transformational. When I saw the engraving of the path to deepest transformation, I realized that my love of cooking could lead me to the answer I had been looking for all along, to overcome that mental and emotional plateau.

1

Alchemy and the Path to "Deepest Transformation"

Alchemy is an ancient practice with a secretive, mysterious reputation. In part, alchemy was a forerunner of chemistry, and it's commonly associated with ancient alchemists' efforts to transform base metals into gold. But the goals of alchemy went much deeper than that. The processes of alchemical transformation—calcination, dissolution, separation, conjunction, fermentation, distillation, and coagulation—were symbols of steps on the path to personal and spiritual transformation, as well. Today, the potential power of alchemy is still expansive, and it is available for us to harness.

When most people think about health, they think about their body, their physiology, about seeing the doctor and about how well various organs are performing. Most people don't see that emotional balance and intellectual stimulation are just as important as a clean bill of physical health. They also think that changing their diet is the key to changing their health, and can't understand why they can't stick to their new healthy eating plans after revamping what they eat. But the big picture of health is more like a puzzle, with many interlocking pieces, and changing your eating habits is just part of the healing equation.

Through my practice of alchemy, I discovered that optimal health is about seeing the connections among the puzzle pieces, and nourishing those pieces so they can fit together quickly, in turn strengthening the pieces of your life, in a natural way that flows. Optimal health is only achieved when these core components are properly balanced in relationship to one another, and food and cooking provide the perfect gateway into this practice.

As I started to practice what I learned from alchemy, some amazing things happened. I totally revamped the way I meditate based on alchemy theory, explored different styles of mediation, and even practiced meditation in nonconventional ways (for example, while standing in line at the grocery store). At the time, I had been feeling physically tired on a regular basis. I'd had a health checkup, but my blood work was normal. I was hoping that meditation would help me to accept that I was just getting older, and that the tiredness was part of it. But one day during a deep meditation, the idea that I should go gluten-free to feel better came to me very strongly—I practically heard it. I followed the urge without question, even though I had already tested negative for both celiac disease and gluten sensitivity. Three weeks later, after removing glutinous foods, I saw a huge improvement in my energy, my skin, and even my waistline.

Shortly afterward, I spoke with Dr. Tom O'Bryan, a well-known gastroenterologist who is also a functional medicinal guru and discovered that my "meditation message" may have been very much on track. As it turns out, standard gluten tests check for only one of the eight proteins people can be sensitive to—not to mention, he said, that anyone with any kind of digestive disorder like mine (IBS) should eliminate gluten permanently. But it was more than a simple question of diet: At the same time I removed gluten from my diet, I had also cultivated a sensual connection with food, using my meal preparation as a healing ritual, and started adding more healing herbs and spices to my meals (even my morning coffee!).

Continuing this integrated practice led me to the approach I now use in my own life and with my health coaching clients. It is impossible to address physical symptoms without also addressing the emotional and spiritual aspects of our health struggles. Physics tells us that all humans (and all things) are made up of energy, and we have to mold and shape this energy. The human "energy engine" is made of seven cylinders (sometimes called chakras), which are important energy centers starting at the top of the head and going down to the base of the spine. These cylinders house all our important glands and organs, from our brain and heart to our stomach and reproductive organs. These centers also correlate to emotions (soul) and our connection to the divine creator force (spirit). Throughout history, most spiritual traditions have talked about the human trinity of body, soul, and spirit and the seven cylinders (yes, even Christianity; Jesus calls them the "seven candles"), but they approach them in different ways. Some have seen certain parts of the trinity or seven cylinders as sinful, or things we should ignore. Alchemists take a totally different approach. For your body to function properly, physically and emotionally, to be "driving" at 100 percent capacity, you must have an even flow of energy to all cylinders, on all three levels. Superfood alchemy is your tool to support your health using this holistic, balanced approach.

Superfood Alchemy: The Transformational Power of Plant Foods

Foods, especially plant foods, are the ideal starting point to grasping the powerful alchemical concept of healing on three levels. Food can be a path to healing in every way: providing basic fuel for the body, supporting mental functioning, and sometimes even appealing to our emotional self with comfort, sensual delight, or a reconnection with nature. In terms of healing, plant foods can go even deeper. They are natural sources of vitamins, minerals, fiber, and fats, and certain plant ingredients contain compounds that work as potent medicine in our body and mind. There is an overwhelming amount of research that plant-based eating can prevent and even reverse disease, and that simply by following a plant-based diet we can address a variety of chronic conditions, such as cancer, heart disease, diabetes, and more. Hippocrates's famous edict, "Let food be thy medicine," is sage advice today! However, to optimize the healing process, certain foods are stronger medicine than others. My goal is to teach you to cook like an alchemist: the recipes in this book incorporate superfoods, medicinal plants, and adaptogens that are known to support healing. By combining and cooking them in specific ways, you can amp up the healing properties of the dish.

3

Before we get any further into the book, there's a lot of misunderstanding about what constitutes a superfood, and you may have never heard of adaptogens, so here's a brief explanation. Superfoods are natural foods, many of them plants, which are packed with nutrients. Compared to other natural foods, they deliver far more powerful doses of the vitamins and minerals you need to maintain energy, heal, and keep feeling good. (For example, 1 cup of kale can provide more than 70% of your RDA for vitamins A, C, and K, plus good levels of fifteen other nutrients, while 1 cup of celery only provides less than 2% to 0% of any one of these nutrients.) Superfoods also contain special plant fibers, pigments, and other protective antioxidants that detoxify various organ systems.

Plants that fall into the category of medicinal plants, such as chamomile, mugwort, and aloe vera, are often not used in a culinary fashion but have been traditionally administered through teas and tinctures by folk healers and alchemists alike. They have been prized for centuries for active chemical compounds that can bring about changes in the body or in certain organ systems, or just to improve immunity. These compounds are produced by plants as defense against natural enemies, including insects, fungi, and herbivorous animals, heat, wind, and other environmental factors. Adaptogens, meanwhile, are the rock stars of the medicinal plant world. They contain special compounds that are unique to each plant. Adaptogens encourage full-body homeostasis (balance) because they are immunity-modulating, meaning they can calm stress

or provide more energy, whichever is needed at that time. Such adaptogens as turmeric, reishi mushroom, and rhodiola not only boost brain performance (that's why these herbs are used prevalently by bio-hackers), but they are beneficial for the neuroendocrine system (how your nervous system communicates with your glands). In helping balance two very important stress hormones, adrenaline and cortisol, adaptogens provide a key to keeping calm, a healthy metabolism, a proper sleep cycle, and countless other functions.

If all of this sounds too medicinal, fear not: In addition to health coaching, I'm a chef and cookbook author, remember? Although these recipes incorporate superfoods and healing plants, they are also delicious, and intended to offer you a tasty, easy way to get these superstar ingredients into your daily routine.

ALCHEMICAL OPERATIONS

Each chapter focuses on one of the seven energy centers in the body and one of the seven operations that are part of the alchemical transformation process. What makes alchemy unique from other mind-body practices is the way in which alchemists approach working with the vital energy centers of the body. Alchemists called their mind-body practice the "Great Work" (which is working on yourself!) and the ways they work on these energy centers are called "operations" (which are also in the titles of the chapters of this book). This book progresses from the first energy center in Chapter 1, Calcination (page 17), where your colon is located, up to your head and brain where the pineal gland is located in Chapter 7, Solidification (page 205). Alchemists are the ultimate holistic healing multitaskers since they believe that nothing is separate and everything is part of a whole. Imbedded in the name of each operation are instructions on how to boost healing or strengthen each energy center—not only on organ/gland level, but also on the soulful and spiritual level as well. If you ever seek out old alchemy texts, you may see laboratory and chemistry-like terminology, since ancient alchemists used coded language in their writing to protect themselves from persecution. Some of them were in fact early chemists or metallurgists, but when they used these laboratory terms, they had double meanings that described work on the self. To alchemists, *you* are your very own laboratory to experiment on to achieve vibrant health and greater purpose in your life. Even if you don't consider yourself a full-blown alchemist, taking some practices from alchemy and incorporating them into your routine can offer a path to better health, clearer thinking, increased energy, and a deeper sense of well-being.

As you work with these recipes, you can as also think of your home, or a combo of your kitchen and living area, as your own "Superfood Alchemy laboratory," where you can enjoy your work with soulful meals, essential oil preparations, and meditation practice. Worried that this will turn into a juggling act? Don't! You have most of the tools for transformation already at your fingertips; it's just about bringing a little more awareness into the equation and following the chapters as your guide to help you along the way.

5

HOW TO USE THIS BOOK

You can work your way through the chapters in this book in the order they are presented, or you can jump around according to your own needs. If you were a coaching client, we'd work on your weakest energy center first to give you a more stable base on your journey toward a healthier you. How do you know which energy center needs healing without having me diagnose you in person? Looking at your physical ailments as a guide for the best place to start. Having tummy troubles? Definitely check out Chapter 3, Separation, to first make sure your digestion is on track. Is your thyroid sluggish? Then Chapter 5, Fermentation, is the ticket. Or perhaps you are feeling brain fog; hop over to Chapter 6. As you nosh your way to a more plant-based, nutrient-rich diet, also begin to incorporate the soulful essential oil therapies for that energy center and support the healing process with meditation work feature at the end of each chapter.

You can certainly thumb through the pages of this book and pick out recipes that strike your fancy or dabble with the meditations, but this book is a manual, intended to fast-track your health holistically through alchemical cooking and living. The more you focus in on specific energy centers to remedy particular imbalances in the threefold body, soul, and spirit way, the stronger the effects will be. So, as you delve into one chapter's delicious food recipe, set an intention to also try the essential oil preparations and the meditations presented in that same chapter. They echo the teaching lessons and give you additional ways to heal in that area. While you may not be able to practice them all in tandem every day, follow the suggestions on how to sneak these practices into even the busiest lifestyle, as I do.

Once you work on the energy center that needs more TLC, you'll want work your way through other chapters, not only to enjoy the delicious recipes and feel good about eating well, but also as a way to strengthen other energy centers and give yourself a broader, more complete nutritional base and culinary variety, while cleaning up your beauty routine, and finding more comfort with your meditation practice.

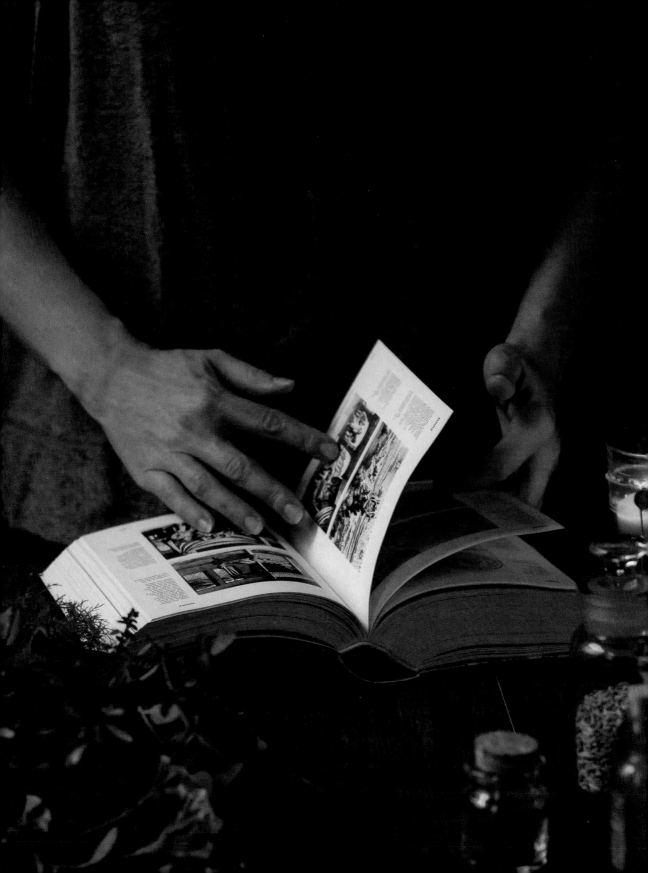

For a more complete alchemy diagnosis, take the online superfood alchemy quiz at www.superfoodalchemy.com/quiz.

Basics of Nutrition

The recipes in this book are based on the healing power of plants. The introduction to each chapter describes how superfoods, healing herbs, and oils carry compounds that can boost healing for a particular energy center. The recipes are plant-based, and most have easy substitutions to customize to your preferred way of eating, whether that's vegetarian, vegan, pescatarian, flexitarian, or Paleo. While the recipes themselves contain no animal proteins, many of them would pair well with grass-fed meats or organic pasture-raised poultry. If you do eat animal protein, sourcing it from a farm that has grass-fed meat is not only better for you (since animals that are grass-fed contain far more omega-3s just as with their dairy), but these farms also tend to treat their animals with more care and respect.

If you are vegetarian who eats dairy, grass-fed sources of dairy are best, as they contain far more omega-3s compared to grain-fed counterparts. Grass-fed dairy can be difficult to find, but if you are fortunate to live within a few hours radius of any grass-fed farm, many of them deliver or may also be part of a CSA (community supported agriculture) service that delivers fresh seasonal produce weekly or monthly. Grass-fed butter is easier to find and is listed throughout the recipes; often, you can swap it for a plant oil if you prefer. You can feel good about using grass-fed butter,

though, since it's not only high in omega-3s and carries a lot of flavor, but is also rich in vitamin D.

If you include eggs in your diet, they are one of the most nutritious foods around and are very beneficial for brain health. Try to find organic, pasture-raised eggs, since hens who lay these eggs are fed differently—making their eggs more nutritious as well as humane.

If you are flexitarian, make vegetables the base of every meal (at least 2 cups or more per meal) without eating high quantities of breads and grains.

For Paleo-style eating, simply omit the grains in the recipes and opt for the vegetable noodles or cauliflower rice for any dish that calls for rice or gluten-free pasta. Beans can be substituted with half the amount of nuts or seeds.

Fat counts in these recipes will seem higher to people who are used to the old, low-fat, high-carb eating model, which we now know is very harmful for the brain and other organ systems. Good-quality fats, such as avocado and olive oil, are incredibly healing for your brain and skin, and help keep hunger and snacking in check since they are so filling. Most nutritionists will also cite 50 to 60 grams of healthy fat per day as acceptable, even with older nutritional models. While this book does not follow a low-carb or ketogenic diet, you'll find more of a balance between healthy fats and better-quality carbs found in vegetables and whole unprocessed grains, which makes the recipes filling while being more moderate in calories.

The recipes were created to be 100 percent gluten-free—although if you can eat gluten, feel free to swap in organic glutinous versions of the pastas and grain products referenced. Recent studies have shown that gluten is extremely problematic for some and moderately problematic for many. If you do decide to eat gluten, go organic whenever possible, since wheat is one of the largest crops in the United States and sprayed with Roundup that contains glyphosate, which is detrimental for gut health and for the gut flora that rule your immune system. There is also a correlation between glyphosate, used in conventional farming, and the massive increase in celiac disease.

Nuts and seeds are included in this book, since they are incredibly healing for your nervous system, brain, and other organs in the body. If you have allergies or an autoimmune condition that precludes consuming nuts or seeds, your doctor may recommend an AIP (autoimmune protocol) diet, which could allow you to reintroduce them later. Alternatively, you can swap out nuts and some seeds in favor of chickpeas. For example, in the roasted nuts with coffee recipe, you can easily use drained, canned chickpeas in place of the mixed nuts. Sesame seeds can be replaced by sunflower seeds or even cooked quinoa.

Nightshade plants, which include tomatoes, potatoes, eggplant, and peppers, are used in the book as well. Like nuts and seeds, these can be problematic for those with an autoimmune illness, in particular psoriasis and rheumatoid arthritis. I suggest working with an integrative or functional medicine physician who is knowledgeable about nutrition and diet to recommend the appropriate plan for you. Enjoy the many recipes in the book that don't contain nightshades.

Soulful Preparations with Essential Oils

Each chapter contains recipes for nonedible products using that chapter's key essential oils. These recipes can be the basis for soulful practices and rituals, including ways to pamper, maintain, boost, and protect your body using essential oil preparations. Soulful practices are meant for relaxation and reconnecting with your body in a soulful yet *mindless* way, to "just be." Use the practices as a way to empty your mind and feel comfortable in your own skin, the ideal prep to calm yourself before meditation. They will also help detoxify your beauty care regimen and replace general toiletries that can be high in toxic ingredients.

Essential oils are featured heavily in this book since they are considered the soul of the plant, capturing the compounds that carry the health benefits and the scent or "personality." Ancient alchemists knew that scents have the power to boost emotions, which could help their patients heal faster. Now, we know that essential oils contain antibacterial, antifungal compounds and are generally a safe way

9

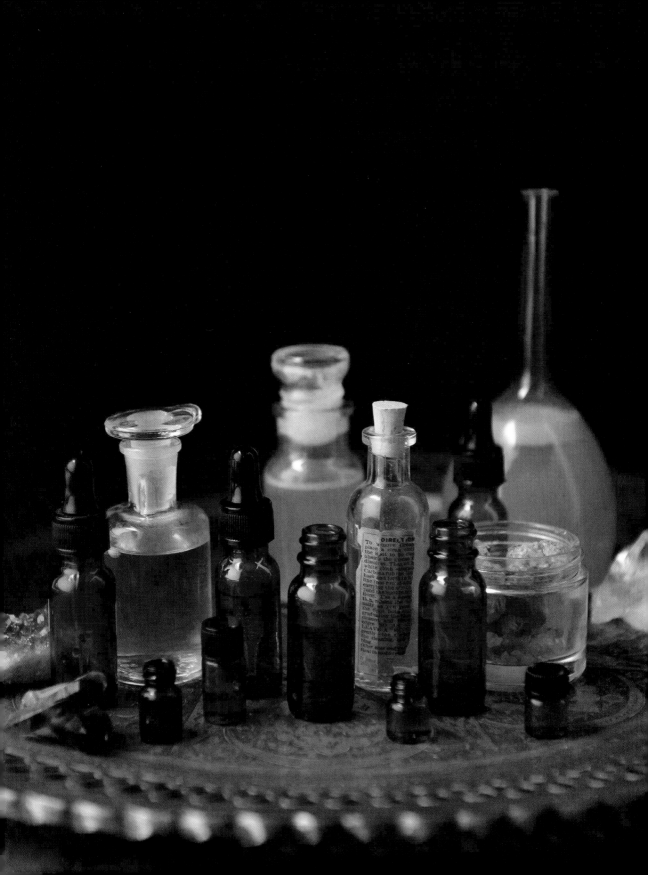

to boost immunity. Modern MDs are catching on to the healing benefits of essential oils used both topically and internally, and almost all integrated physicians prescribe essential oils as a therapy to be combined with other healing modalities, such as food and exercise.

Since each essential oil has a distinct odor and character, they also resonate more strongly with specific energy centers, just like the superfoods featured, which is why they are assigned to specific chapters. However, many of these oils can be used in tandem with each other regardless of their assigned chapter and you may find that they have multiple benefits (just like the super-foods) to bring healing and enjoyment.

Essential Oil Basics

Essential oils vary greatly in quality. Typically, the higher the quality, the higher the price and the more aromatic the oil. Essential oils can be pricey since it takes pounds of plant materials, including flowers, stems, leaves, and roots, to produce the oils. If you're on a tight budget, you can still indulge in some essential oils, such as lemon, orange, lime, basil, rosemary, oregano, and black pepper; those plants are cheaper and more prevalently grown, so their oils can be found for a lower price.

Once you purchase your first set of oils, find a dark, dry, cool cabinet to store them in, away from sunlight or heat that can turn the oils rancid. Be judicious about choosing oils, since they last for months and up to one year. Great starter oils, that

you will most likely make the most use of, include lavender, frankincense, orange, and cardamom. Not all oils are safe to use directly from the bottle topically (such as cinnamon, which can burn), so follow the instructions listed in each essential oil preparation, or consult the essential oil company guide before applying oils directly to skin.

Lavender and frankincense are typically well tolerated straight from the bottle, but you can always test them on the inside of your forearm first for interactions. If you have a food allergy, steer clear of the oils made from those foods. Essential oils are not always safe for infants, children, and pets, so consult your doctor or veterinarian before using them or even diffusing oils in your home. Some essential oils are safe to eat, but they must be food grade, so check with the manufacturer, and note that just a few drops will flavor an entire dish. If you're on prescription medication, check with your doctor before ingesting essential oils or herbs, as they may have drug interactions.

An essential oil diffuser is a smart purchase and a way to enjoy your collection of essential oils daily; it's required for all the diffuser blends in this book. Look for brands that are labeled "ultrasonic" since they produce a heavier mist and help humidify the air as they scent.

Meditations

Because a holistic approach to wellness is a core component of alchemy, each chapter ends with one or two simple meditations.

Daily rituals can help you to feel grounded; beyond healthy eating, meditation is another practice that you can adopt to live a more intentional life. Countless studies have shown that meditation has serious benefits for your body, including blood pressure control and improved sleep, and it can even facilitate better eating habits and weight loss. If you are not meditating regularly already, I hope you'll start now.

Consider meditation a new skill to be developed. It's crucial to maintain a positive attitude and be patient with yourself while learning meditation. Think of it this way: treat yourself as the child version of you, learning to ride a bike for the first time. Be patient, calm, and supportive to yourself as you learn this new challenging skill, even when you make mistakes. If you're a first timer, I recommend trying a few different meditations first to get a feel for it, and then focusing in on the meditation practice for the energy center you want to rebalance. For newbies and seasoned meditation pros alike, I also suggest beginning your meditation practice with a simple shielding visualization exercise (see Meditation Preparation, page 239). Meditation can sometimes bring up strong feelings, so this exercise will help you to feel relaxed and comfortable as you progress into deeper states (for more on brain waves during meditation, see page 237).

Making meditation part of your daily routine is easier when you pick the same time of day to meditate. Find a quiet place to practice for the first month or two.

Most of the practices in this book can be completed in ten minutes or less, but as you progress, you can increase your time, try different styles, and try meditating in other locations. Once you become more disciplined, you'll find you'll be easily able to meditate in noisier environments (even on public transportation—one of my favorite places to meditate!) and go into a calm mode more quickly than ever before.

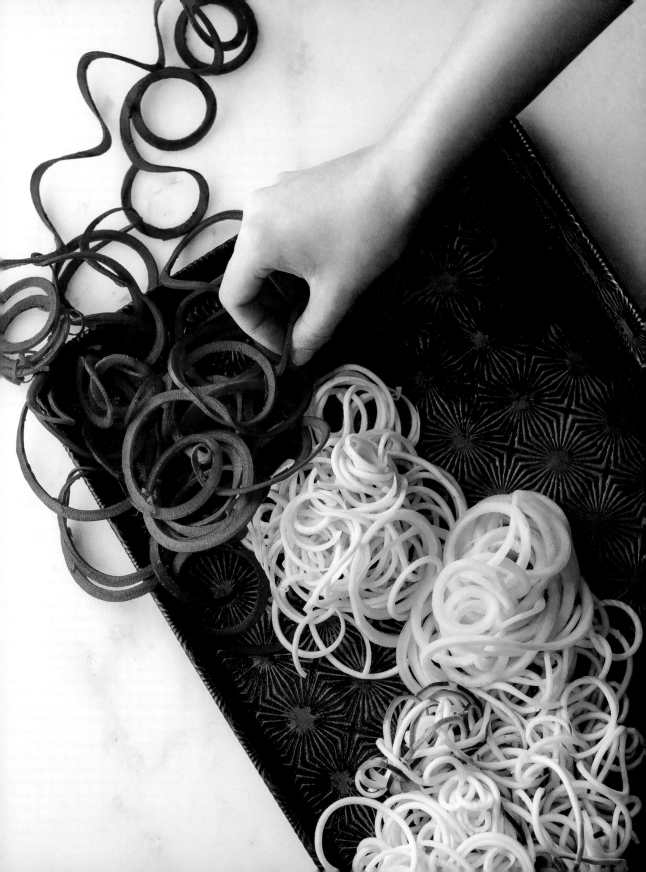

OUTFITTING THE SUPERFOOD ALCHEMY LAB

Essential Kitchen Tools

Beyond the basics—pots and pans, cutting boards, and a good kitchen knife—I recommend adding these kitchen tools to your supply to get cooking like an alchemist.

MORTAR AND PESTLE: A mortar and pestle is an old-fashioned alchemy and apothecary tool for grinding herbs, spices, and salt. It will allow you to be more hands-on with the recipes and preparations in this book. Fresh-grinding your ingredients makes whole spices more flavorful and potent and makes them easier to digest. Shop for a mortar and pestle in discount housewares stores. Since alchemical cooking is all about making food a sensual experience, buy whatever material delights your eyes, be it granite, marble, or even copper. (If you don't have a mortar and pestle, you can use a heavy skillet or a pepper mill to crack black peppercorns, but don't use pre-ground black pepper; it loses its essential oils and flavor as it sits.)

CAST-IRON COOKWARE: I recommend using cast-iron cookware for many recipes. As a Superfood Alchemy tool, it does double duty. Cast-iron cookware creates more flavor by helping brown your food better, since cast iron captures more heat. And what's more, cooking with cast iron adds mineral iron to your diet.

CAST-IRON ROUND DUTCH OVEN: Dutch ovens hold heat better and are less likely to burn delicate foods. This is the only heavy-duty pot that you'll ever need to pull off gently melting chocolate without a double boiler and working with delicate essential oil preparations that clean up fast. They come in many sizes; a 1- to 2-quart Dutch oven is generally suitable for families of one or two, and larger sizes up to 9 quarts are good for a large family. A 1-quart Dutch oven is what I recommend for the essential oil recipes. If you can manage it, I think such brands as Le Creuset are well worth the investment.

VEGETABLE NOODLE MAKER: "I have trouble getting more pasta into my diet," said no one anywhere ever. A vegetable noodle maker or spiralizer is a great way to satisfy two needs, your craving for pasta and your desire to eat more vegetables, with one tool. Most noodle makers are inexpensive and are dishwasher safe. They are so simple to use and even the most intimidated new kitchen alchemist can use it: just insert the blade, add the veggie, and turn the crank!

MICROPLANE: All kitchen alchemists have a few tools they feel they just can't do without, and this is one of mine! A fine-toothed Microplane produces fine, uniform shavings of the toughest spices and heartiest nuts, from whole cloves to nutmeg and Brazil nuts, to top your meals with garnishes that have a fluffy texture and healing benefits. Microplanes make for fast cleanup, too, since they are slender and don't take up much space in your dishwasher or sink!

TEA INFUSER OR STRAINER: You can boost flavor and healing in your cooking by incorporating brewed teas into soups, smoothies, sauces, and more. (Not to mention, you can get creative making your own tea blends to sip and savor!) Many of the teas that are featured in this cookbook can be purchased in tea bag form, but if you're buying loose teas, which can be a lot more economical, you may want to use a tea infuser or strainer. In a pinch, you can also brew the leaves directly in the water and strain before using, or fashion your own tea bags from cheesecloth.

PLASTIC OR GLASS MEASURING CUP WITH SPOUT: Shop for a PBP-free plastic or glass measuring cup that can be dedicated to all the essential oil preparations in this book—I recommend having a separate measuring cup to use for nonedible preparations. If you don't mind scratches and a little left over wax, a plastic cup can simply be wiped out with paper towels after essential oil preparations—perfect for the lazier alchemist! If you are a neat freak, use glass, and clean beeswax from it with boiling water.

15

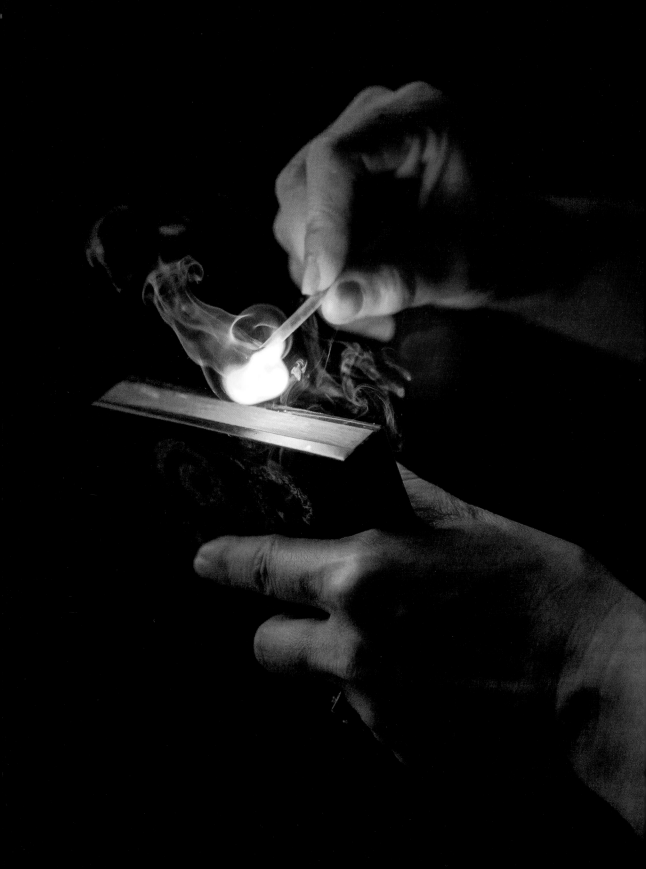

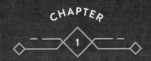

CHAPTER 1

Calcination

FEELING THE BURN, DETOXING THE BODY

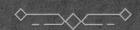

Calcination is the fiery alchemical operation associated with purification or "detox."

Do you feel as though your health and your life hasn't lived up to your expectations? Do you find that negative thinking keeps you from moving closer to your goals and attaining the things you are meant to have in your life? Then, this chapter can help. Unclear, negative thinking and low moods can be a factor of diet (as you'll discover in Chapter 7), but we live in a very toxic modern age; every day, we are exposed to environmental toxins, whether from pollution, leakage of heavy metals in our waterways and farmlands, or even the clothes and cosmetics we wear. Cleaning up your act through detox can fast-track your healing on many levels at once. The recipes and preparations for calcination will help you to release toxins *and* old ways of thinking that you just don't need. The best way to detox is to make the decision to do so, then take action on all levels: body, soul, and spirit. Your body and mind both have the innate ability to adapt and heal, and detox may help these processes along.

Calcination is the fiery alchemical operation associated with purification or detox. The recipes and therapies in this chapter correspond to the base energy center surrounding the colon, part of the large intestines through which you eliminate waste. If you want to be stricter with the detox, juice in the morning, then stick to the nondairy options for the recipes and avoid nonvegan sources of protein for five to ten days to boost your body's ability to cleanse. You can also try intermittent fasting, eating in a specific eight-hour window, a great way to rest your digestive system and limit calories.

Superfoods, Herbs, and Essential Oils for Detox

ROOTS AND ALLIUMS (CARROTS, BEETS, ONIONS, AND GARLIC): These foods are naturally healing for the base energy center, also sometimes called the root chakra. Starchy tubers have a special kind of starch, called resistant starch, which gut microbes ferment into many healing, colon-friendly compounds.

BLACK PEPPERCORNS AND BLACK PEPPER ESSENTIAL OIL: Black peppercorns heat up your dishes and help you feel the burn while supercharging detox. Black pepper contains the alkaloid compound piperine, which has been associated with cancer prevention and, when paired up with medicinal foods, such as turmeric, drastically increases the absorption of the other's detoxifying compounds. Black peppercorns in your grocer's spice aisle can be pricey, but you will get them for a steal if you purchase them in bulk online or at a natural food store.

CAYENNE PEPPER: This little flame-shaped chile gives a fruity heat to dishes. Capsaicin, the active component in cayenne, is a fiery fierce detox partner: it revs up your heart, and in turn your metabolic rate, for faster calorie burn, and may even help boost energy with faster fat breakdown.

NETTLE: Used widely by the ancient Egyptians and Romans for muscle and joint pain, this prickly plant (also known as stinging nettle) is a soothing tonic in disguise since its "painful" active compounds actually quench inflammation. The leaves of stinging nettle can be brewed as a delicious dark green tea, without feeling the effects of their stinging hairs or needles.

RHODIOLA ROOT: This prized adaptogen, valued by herbalists for improving both mental and physical fatigue, is currently being studied since it may lower cortisol (the stress hormone) with its unique blend of antioxidants and antibacterial compounds.

CEDARWOOD ESSENTIAL OIL: Cedarwood is used to help you feel supported, a definite plus during the detoxifying process. Cedarwood oil can add a spa-like scent to your home, since saunas are built from cedar.

VETIVER ESSENTIAL OIL: Lush, grassy, and lemony, vetiver is used to calm "toxic thinking" that brings on emotional stress and in one small study has shown to be helpful for sounder sleep.

Want a tasty drink that'll also give you an overall boost to tackle the day? This recipe contains rhodiola root, an adaptogen that may help ward off fatigue as it burns fat. Beets are high in natural nitrates, which can boost your energy and regulate metabolism.

Beet Almond Smoothie
WITH RHODIOLA ROOT

SERVES 2

2 small beets (about ½ pound)

1 cup brewed rhodiola tea

⅔ cup vanilla protein powder or plain Greek yogurt

½ cup coconut milk

¼ cup almonds

½ teaspoon almond extract

1 teaspoon stevia (optional)

Wash the beets and trim off the ends; no need to peel them. Grate them on a box grater and transfer them to a blender. Add the tea, protein powder, coconut milk, almonds, almond extract, and stevia (if using). Blend until smooth, then serve immediately in two glasses.

per serving
224 *calories*
9 g (3 g) *fat (sat)*
18 g *carbs*
10 g *sugar*
7 g *fiber*
22 g *protein*
158 mg *sodium*

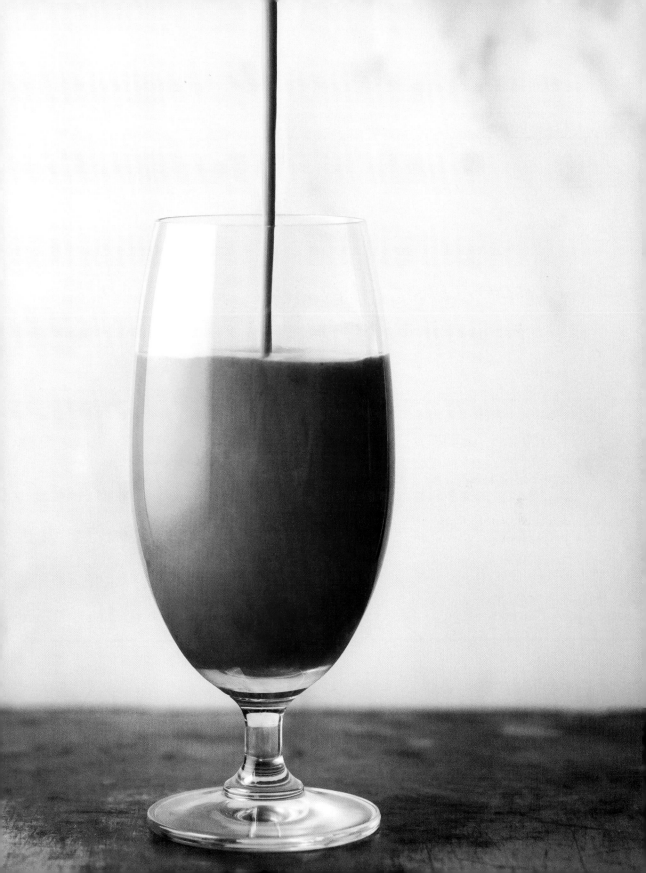

If you like guacamole, you'll adore this avocado-centric, savory smoothie that also makes a fantastic snack or less sweet breakfast. If you don't have lime on hand, you can easily substitute lemon. Using nettle tea in your smoothie in place of milk not only ramps up the antioxidant load, but allows you to flirt with herbalism in the simplest way possible, by making this healing herb tea part of your breakfast.

Herbalism Green Smoothie
WITH NETTLE TEA

SERVES 2

2 cups packed spinach

1 cup brewed nettle tea

½ cucumber

2 celery stalks

1 avocado, pitted and peeled

Juice of ½ lemon

2 tablespoons chopped fresh cilantro or basil

1 teaspoon fresh thyme leaves (optional)

8 ice cubes

Place the spinach, tea, cucumber, celery, avocado, lemon juice, cilantro or basil, thyme (if using), and ice cubes in a blender. Process until smooth and divide between two glasses. Serve immediately.

NOTE: To brew the tea, pour 1 cup of boiling water over one nettle leaf tea bag or 1 tablespoon of dried nettle leaves in an infuser. Steep for at least 10 minutes; the longer you let it steep, the stronger the tea will be (some people recommend infusing nettle for several hours, so you could even steep the tea overnight so it's ready to go in the morning). Let cool completely before using in this recipe.

per serving
211 *calories*
16 g (3 g) *fat (sat)*
19 g *carbs*
6 g *sugar*
10 g *fiber*
5 g *protein*
60 mg *sodium*

Fight fire (inflammation) with fire (hot chiles)! Hot peppers cause a thermogenic reaction in your body, which can boost calorie burn for up to 30 minutes after you eat them. They are also a wonderful detox helper, since they are naturally low in calories, aid with weight loss, and contain detoxifying nutrients, including vitamin C.

HOT CHILE ANTI-INFLAMMATION AND
Weight-Loss Shot

SERVES 8

Place the coconut water, cherries, habanero pepper, and cinnamon in a blender. Blend until smooth. Divide among eight shot glasses and serve immediately.

1 cup coconut water

½ cup frozen cherries or raspberries

½ habanero pepper, seeded; 1 jalapeño pepper, chopped; or 1 teaspoon cayenne powder

Pinch of ground cinnamon

per serving
11 *calories*
0 g (0 g) *fat (sat)*
2 g *carbs*
2 g *sugar*
1 g *fiber*
0 g *protein*
32 mg *sodium*

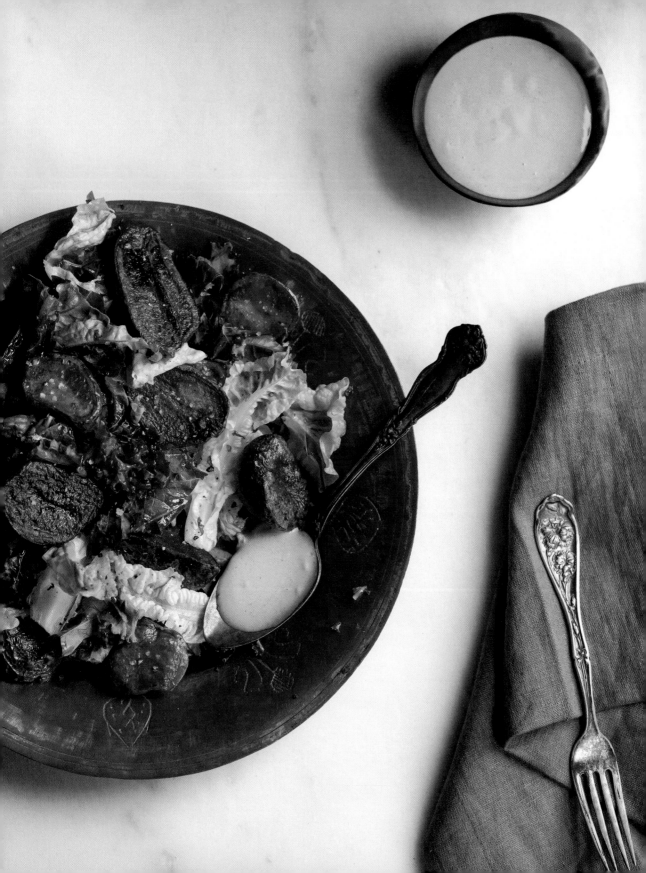

Feeling chilly, but still crave a salad? Cozy up with this nutrient-packed one-skillet dish that's rich in vitamin K for bone health and iron for heart health. The sriracha turns up the heat while adding the active chile compound capsaicin, an important antioxidant that is also a tumor preventative.

Hot Winter Kale Potato Salad
WITH SRIRACHA MAYO DRIZZLE

SERVES 4

¼ cup mayonnaise or vegan mayonnaise

1 to 2 tablespoons sriracha

1 tablespoon tomato paste

2 tablespoons olive oil

1 pound creamer or small purple Peruvian potatoes, cut in half

½ teaspoon salt

¼ teaspoon freshly ground black pepper

1 pound baby kale, trimmed

Place the mayonnaise in a small bowl along with the sriracha, tomato paste, and 1 tablespoon of warm water. Whisk well and set aside.

Heat the olive oil in a skillet, preferably cast iron, over medium heat. Add the potatoes, cut side down, and cook, turning occasionally, for 12 to 15 minutes, or until they start to brown. Sprinkle with the salt and pepper and cook for 5 minutes more, or until they are fork-tender. Transfer to a plate. Add the kale to the hot skillet and cook, turning often, for 5 to 7 minutes, or until the kale is tender. Transfer the kale to the plate with the potatoes. Drizzle with the mayo mixture and serve immediately.

per serving
292 *calories*
18 g (3 g) *fat (sat)*
31 g *carbs*
5 g *sugar*
5 g *fiber*
6 g *protein*
555 mg *sodium*

The aroma of this dish alone, with golden roasted garlic, will entice you to make it again and again. Prized by folk healers as a way to clean from the inside out, garlic actually contains powerful antioxidants that are antibacterial and antifungal. Channel your inner Italian grandmother and stir and sniff often to create the creamy texture this beloved dish is known for.

PAN-ROASTED GARLIC AND CRACKED BLACK PEPPER *Risotto*

SERVES 6

2 quarts vegetable stock

1 tablespoon olive oil

6 whole garlic cloves

1 teaspoon salt

2 tablespoons unsalted grass-fed butter or coconut oil

2 cups uncooked short-grain white risotto rice, such as Arborio or Carnaroli

1 medium-size onion, chopped

½ teaspoon plus ¼ teaspoon freshly ground black pepper

1 tablespoon heavy cream or coconut cream

½ cup grated Parmesan cheese, or ¼ cup nutritional yeast

Heat the stock in a medium-size saucepan over medium heat. Meanwhile, heat the olive oil in a large skillet over medium heat. Add the garlic and ½ teaspoon of the salt to the skillet and cook, turning occasionally, for 10 to 15 minutes, or until the garlic turns dark brown and starts to soften. Transfer the garlic to a cutting board and let rest until cool to the touch, about 5 minutes. Roughly chop the garlic, then return it to the skillet and add the butter.

Add the rice and onion to the skillet with the garlic and place over medium heat. Sprinkle with the remaining ½ teaspoon of salt and ½ teaspoon of the pepper. Cook for 2 to 3 minutes, stirring well to coat the rice.

Add a few cups of the heated stock and bring to a simmer over medium heat. Stir the rice occasionally, adding more broth by ladlefuls as the level of the broth dips below the level of the rice. Cook for 20 to 25 minutes, or until you have added all the stock, most of the liquid is absorbed, and the rice kernels are fairly tender with a slightly firm texture in the center of the grain. Turn off the heat and let rest for 2 minutes. Add the cream and Parmesan (or nutritional yeast) and stir well. Garnish with the remaining ¼ teaspoon of pepper and serve immediately.

1⅓ cups with butter
323 *calories*
10 g (4 g) *fat (sat)*
51 g *carbs*
1 g *sugar*
1 g *fiber*
8 g *protein*
1,638 mg *sodium*

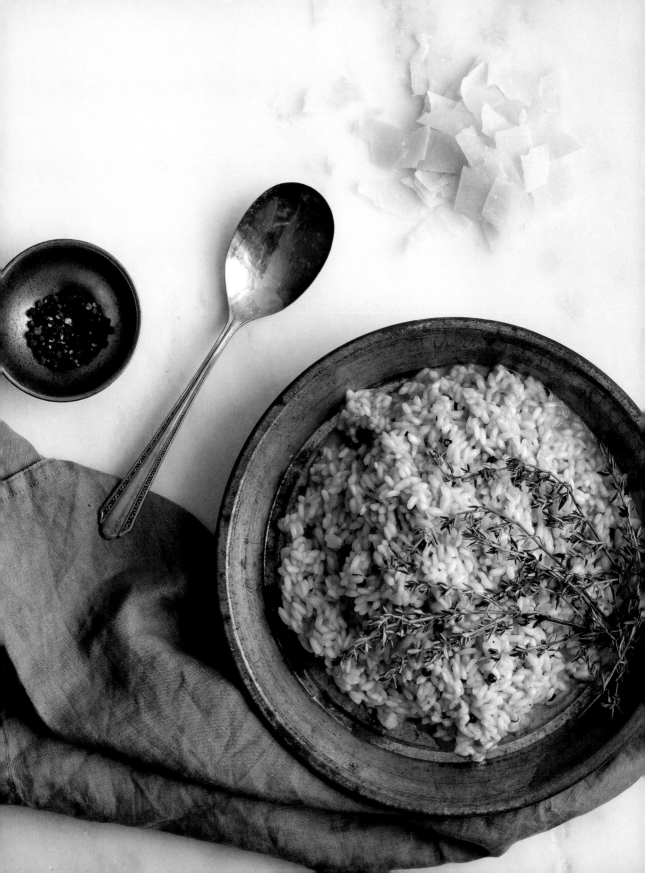

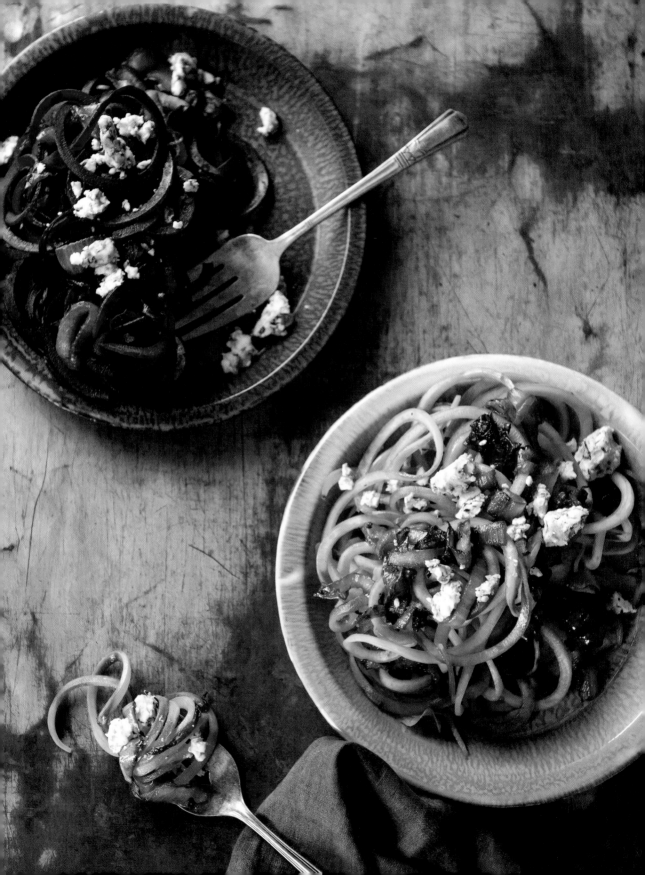

Sweet beets and rich caramelized onions are an irresistible combination. This dish uses a spiralizer to create a fun texture that would be perfect for kids or the big kid in you! Beets contain betaine, a nutrient that may help fight inflammation and protect your cells.

Beet Spaghetti

WITH CARAMELIZED ONIONS AND CRUMBLED FETA

SERVES 4

Using a spiralizer or vegetable noodle maker, process the beets into pasta shapes. Set aside.

Heat the oil in a large skillet over medium heat. Add the onions, salt, and coconut sugar, tossing well. Lower the heat to medium-low and caramelize the onions: cook, stirring occasionally, for 35 to 40 minutes, or until they turn dark brown. Add a few tablespoons of water if the onions start to stick.

When the onions are done, coat another large skillet with cooking spray. Heat over medium heat. Add the beet noodles and cook for 5 to 6 minutes, or until tender. Top with the caramelized onions and toss well. Sprinkle with the crumbled feta and serve immediately.

2 pounds small red or yellow beets, peeled

3 tablespoons olive oil

3 medium-size onions, thinly sliced

½ teaspoon salt

1 tablespoon coconut sugar or honey

Cooking spray

1 cup crumbled feta cheese or cubed silken tofu

— —◇— —
1¼ cups
337 *calories*
18 g (6 g) *fat (sat)*
39 g *carbs*
24 g *sugar*
9 g *fiber*
12 g *protein*
863 mg *sodium*
— —◇— —

Vanilla isn't just relegated to the realm of desserts and pastry; you can also make delicious savory dishes with it, as it adds an almost buttery note. Sweet potatoes are high in vitamin A, which is a necessary nutrient for your top detox organ, the liver. Sweet potatoes are also rich in fiber (6 grams in just 1 cup), a natural cleaner for your intestines and food for your microbiome.

VANILLA-SCENTED
Sweet Potato Soup

SERVES 4

3 tablespoons olive oil or unsalted grass-fed butter

1 small onion, finely chopped

2 garlic cloves, thinly sliced

¼ to ½ teaspoon freshly ground black pepper, plus more for garnish

¼ teaspoon ground cayenne pepper (optional)

1 pound sweet potatoes (about 2 large), peeled and chopped

1 quart vegetable stock

1 teaspoon pure vanilla extract

¼ cup sour cream or coconut cream

Heat the oil in a large stockpot over medium-high heat. Add the onion, garlic, black pepper, and cayenne (if using) and cook for 3 to 5 minutes, or until the onion has softened slightly. Add sweet potatoes and stir to coat with the oil. Add the stock and bring to a boil, then lower heat to a simmer and cover. Simmer for 40 to 45 minutes, or until the sweet potatoes are tender. Remove from the heat and stir in the vanilla. Let cool slightly.

Run the sweet potato mixture through a blender or food processor until well pureed. Alternatively, leave the mixture in the pot and use an immersion blender. If the soup is too thick, add ¼ to ½ cup of water to reach your desired thickness. Garnish with the sour cream or coconut cream and black pepper to taste, then serve immediately.

per serving
263 *calories*
14 g (3 g) *fat (sat)*
27 g *carbs*
6 g *sugar*
4 g *fiber*
8 g *protein*
464 mg *sodium*

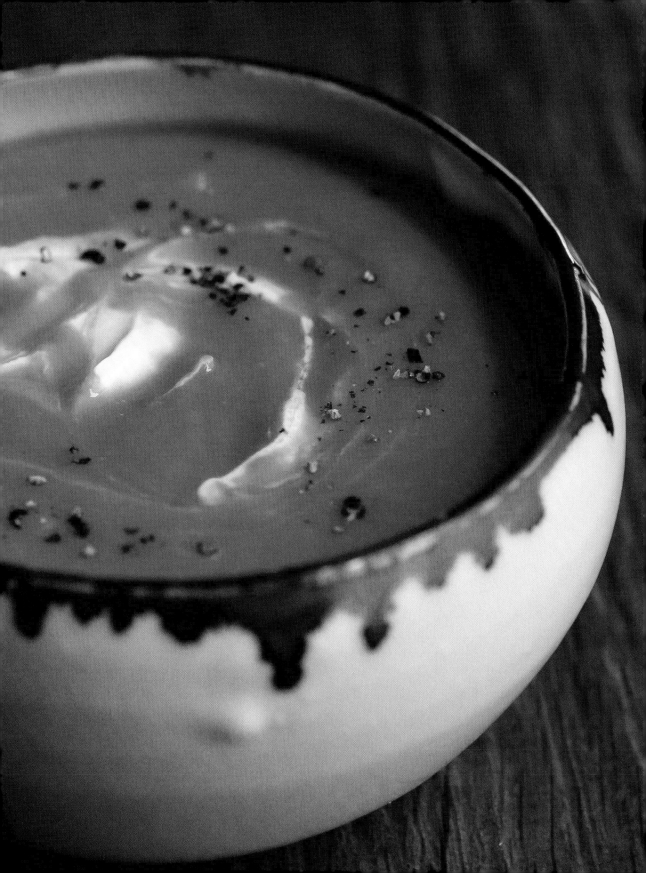

Tangy salt and vinegar potato chips are a salt lover's dream but offer more calories than they do nutrients. To get the most nutrition from this starchier root dish, choose purple potatoes to bring in antioxidants. You can also use smaller potatoes, which are much higher in fiber compared to their large counterparts.

SALT AND VINEGAR
Roasted Purple Potatoes

SERVES 8

2 pounds purple potatoes, or smaller varietals, halved

1 cup plus 2 tablespoons distilled white vinegar

2 teaspoons kosher salt

2 tablespoons unsalted grass-fed butter or olive oil

1 teaspoon freshly ground black pepper

2 tablespoons chopped fresh chives or scallions

Combine the potatoes, 1 cup of the vinegar, and 1 teaspoon of the salt in a medium-size saucepan; add water to cover by 1 inch. Bring to a boil, lower the heat, and simmer until the potatoes are tender, 20 to 25 minutes. Drain and let rest for 5 minutes to allow any water clinging to the potatoes to evaporate.

Heat the butter in a large skillet over medium-high heat. Add the potatoes and season with the remaining 1 teaspoon of salt and the pepper. Cook, turning occasionally, until the potatoes are golden brown and crisp, 10 to 12 minutes. Drizzle with the remaining 2 tablespoons of vinegar. Serve topped with the chives.

— ◇ —
1 cup
122 *calories*
4 g (1 g) *fat (sat)*
18 g *carbs*
2 g *sugar*
3 g *fiber*
2 g *protein*
602 mg *sodium*
— ◇ —

Love beets, but don't relish their long cooking time? Grating them raw is a fast and flavorful way to use them and prep this plant-based ice cream. Naturally sweet superfoods like beets are ideal for detox-friendly desserts. They satisfy your sweet tooth, but are also rich in nutrients, including folate, manganese, and betalains, important for detox. Chocolate is a health food when it contains low amounts of sugar and at least 70% cacao content. If you can't find real dark chocolate chips, buy a 70% bar and chop it.

Beet Orange Ice Cream
WITH DARK CHOCOLATE CHIPS

SERVES 6

Wash the beet and trim the ends. Grate the beet on a box grater and transfer to a blender along with the orange, coconut milk, chocolate chips, and xanthan gum (if using). Blend until smooth. Transfer to an ice-cream machine and process according to the manufacturer's instructions.

If you don't have an ice-cream maker, place the mixture in an airtight container and freeze for 1 hour. Remove from the freezer and scrape the mixture with a fork. Return the container to the freezer and freeze for at least 1 more hour before serving.

*1 medium-size beet
(about 4 ounces)*

1 orange, peeled

1 (14.5-ounce) can coconut milk

½ cup bittersweet chocolate chips

*½ teaspoon xanthan gum
(optional)*

½ cup
219 *calories*
18 g (0 g) *fat (sat)*
14 g *carbs*
10 g *sugar*
2 g *fiber*
2 g *protein*
21 mg *sodium*

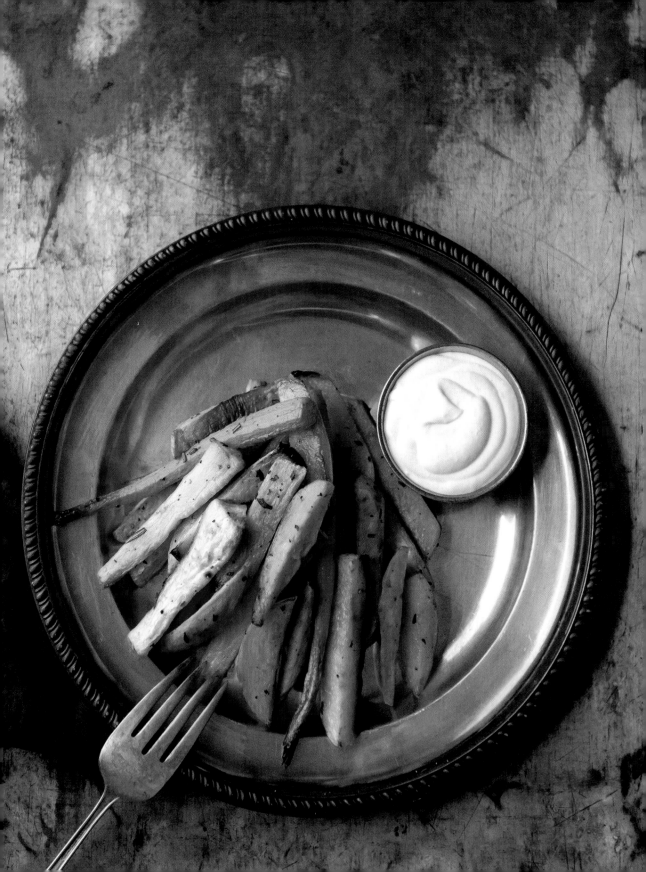

Tempting snacks can sidetrack you from your goal of eating better. This warm vegetable platter is a great option if you find yourself wanting heavy, starchy comfort foods. It pairs root vegetables for detox with a rich-tasting dipping sauce that contains healthy fats for satiety.

ROASTED
Root Vegetable Platter
WITH LEMONY AIOLI

SERVES 6

Preheat the oven to 400°F. Coat two large baking sheets with cooking spray. Place the olive oil in a large bowl along with the rosemary, oregano or thyme, salt, and pepper. Toss the potatoes, celery root, rutabaga, carrots, and parsnips in the olive oil mixture and spread them out on the two prepared baking sheets.

Bake, turning occasionally, for 35 to 40 minutes, or until the vegetables are tender and well browned.

While the vegetables are cooking, prepare the aioli: Place the garlic in a food processor and pulse five or six times to finely chop. Add the mayonnaise and lemon juice and blend again until smooth. Serve with the root vegetables.

Cooking spray

2 tablespoons olive oil

2 tablespoons chopped fresh rosemary

2 tablespoons chopped fresh oregano or thyme

½ teaspoon salt

¼ teaspoon freshly ground black pepper

1 pound red-skinned potatoes or sweet potatoes, unpeeled, scrubbed, and cut into 1-inch pieces

1 pound celery root (celeriac), peeled and cut into 1-inch pieces

1 pound rutabaga, peeled and cut into 1-inch pieces

1 pound carrots, peeled and cut into 1-inch pieces

½ pound parsnips, peeled and cut into 1-inch pieces

2 garlic cloves, peeled

½ cup mayonnaise or vegan mayonnaise

2 tablespoons freshly squeezed lemon juice (from ½ lemon)

per serving
360 *calories*
20 g (3 g) *fat (sat)*
44 g *carbs*
14 g *sugar*
9 g *fiber*
5 g *protein*
487 mg *sodium*

35

If you're craving starchy fries, don't hit the drive-through. Head to your oven to get a tasty, fulfilling lower-carb version: sweet potato and parsnip fries. For a spicier variation, omit the paprika and replace it with an equal amount of chipotle chile powder.

Root Vegetable Fries

SERVES 4

¾ pound parsnips, peeled

¾ pound sweet potatoes, peeled

2 tablespoons olive oil

4 garlic cloves, minced

½ cup grated Parmesan cheese, or ¼ cup nutritional yeast

1 teaspoon paprika

1 teaspoon onion powder

¼ teaspoon ground turmeric

1 teaspoon garlic salt

Preheat the oven to 375°F. Line a baking sheet with a piece of aluminum foil. Cut the parsnips and potatoes into French fry–size sticks, about ⅓ inch by 4 inches. Place in a large bowl along with the olive oil, garlic, Parmesan, paprika, onion powder, turmeric, and garlic salt and toss to coat. Spread out on the prepared baking sheet and bake until the outside is crispy and the inside is tender, 40 to 45 minutes. Serve immediately.

per serving
248 calories
10 g (3 g) fat (sat)
35 g carbs
8 g sugar
7 g fiber
7 g protein
449 mg sodium

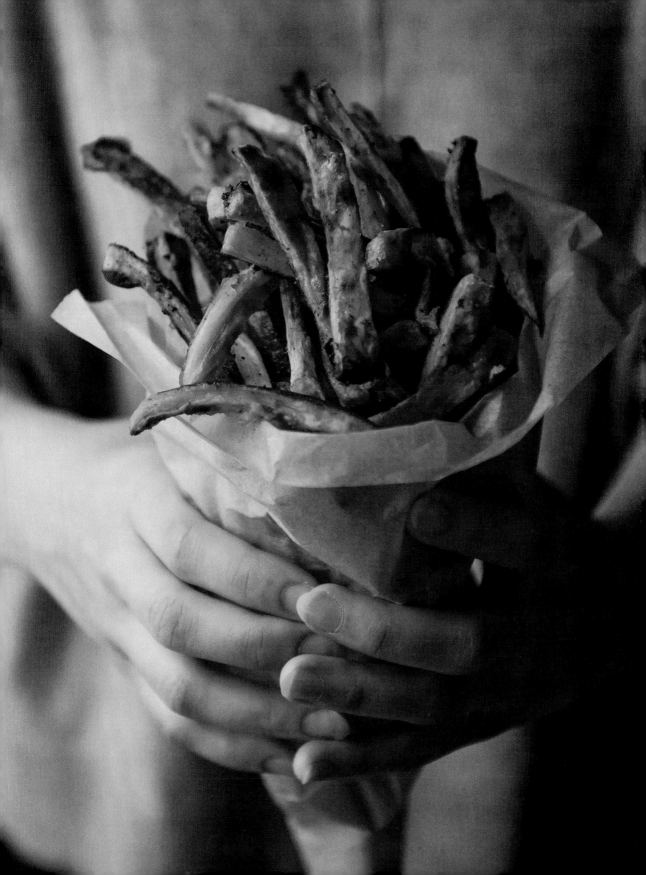

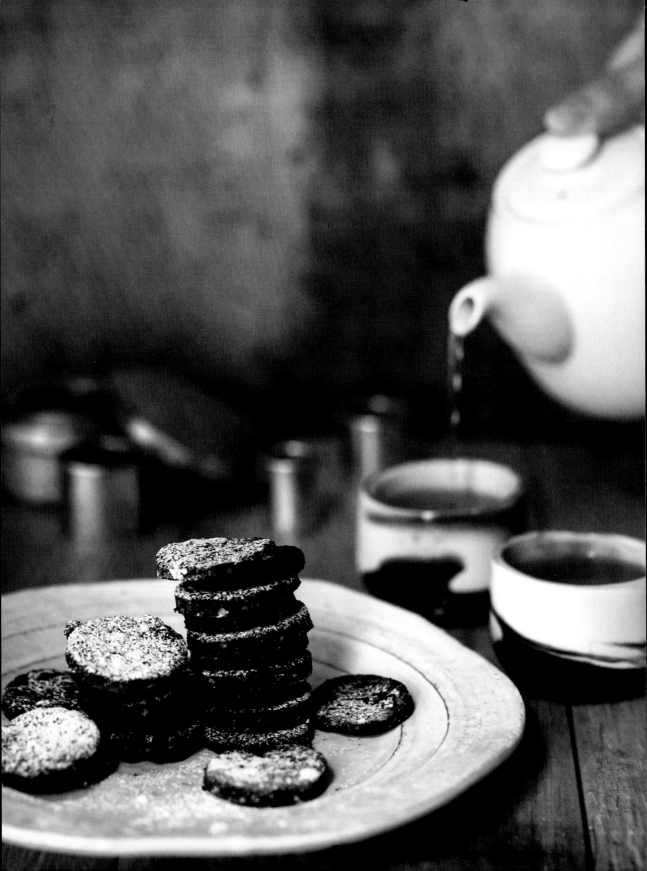

Looking for a sweet treat that won't derail your detox? Then you'll dig these crisp little numbers, which will remind you of an Oreo minus the cream filling. Walnuts are among the healthiest of nuts and offer big doses of fiber, protein, and healthy omega-3 fats, along with antioxidants and various vitamins and minerals. Activated charcoal is an odorless powder that extracts chemicals and toxins from the body; buy food-grade activated charcoal powder online.

ACTIVATED CHARCOAL–INFUSED
Cookies

MAKES 3 DOZEN COOKIES

Place the butter in the freezer for 30 minutes. Meanwhile, preheat the oven to 375°F. Cover a large baking sheet with parchment paper.

In a food processor, combine the frozen butter, flour, walnuts, charcoal, and salt. Process until the walnuts are finely ground into the flour, about 15 seconds.

Add the ice water and pulse briefly, just until the water is distributed evenly and the dough begins to come together in large pieces. Turn out the dough into the counter and sprinkle with a tablespoon of the charcoal to roll it out. Using a round 1-inch cookie cutter, cut out the dough and transfer to a baking sheet, spacing the disks ½ inch apart. Bake for 10 to 15 minutes, or until the edges of the cookies turn golden brown. Transfer to a wire rack to cool completely, then sprinkle with powdered sugar. Serve immediately or store in an airtight container for up to 5 days.

4 tablespoons (½ stick, 4 ounces) unsalted grass-fed butter or vegan butter spread, cubed

1 cup gluten-free multipurpose flour

½ cup walnut pieces

2 tablespoons activated charcoal, plus more to roll the cookies

¼ teaspoon salt

2 to 3 tablespoons ice water

¼ cup powdered sugar

NOTE: When you use activated charcoal internally, be sure to stay extra hydrated to flush everything from your system, and don't use within 2 to 3 hours of taking any prescription medications.

---

2 cookies
49 *calories*
3 g (1 g) *fat (sat)*
3 g *carbs*
0.5 g *sugar*
0 g *fiber*
0.5 g *protein*
18 mg *sodium*

Essential Oil Preparations and Rituals for Calcination

DIFFUSER OIL BLEND FOR FEELING GROUNDED

Vetiver, often used in men's cologne, comes from the roots of a lush grass and has a refreshing herbaceous scent. It is balanced with spicy black pepper in this diffuser blend, which can calm with a hint of heat.

3 drops vetiver oil

2 drops black pepper essential oil

Fill your essential oil diffuser with water according to the diffuser instructions. Add the oils and turn on the mister.

DIFFUSER OIL BLEND FOR FEELING GROUNDED AND UPLIFTED

Black pepper give this blend that smoky, earthy scent that's sweetened up with refreshing orange.

3 drops black pepper essential oil

2 drops orange essential oil

Fill your essential oil diffuser with water according to the diffuser instructions. Add the oils and turn on the mister.

HOMEMADE WET BRUSH EYELINER

We often think of detox in terms of foods and cleanses, but there are external preparations you can use, too. Detoxing your eyeliner is a wise idea since most commercial eyeliners are made with toxic ingredients.

2 teaspoons coconut oil

2 teaspoons aloe vera gel

2 teaspoons activated charcoal

Place the coconut oil, aloe vera gel, and charcoal in a small bowl. Stir well to combine. Using a thin brush, brush on the eyeliner, then allow to dry. Store, refrigerated, for up to 1 month.

ACTIVATED CHARCOAL MASK

When used in moderation, sparkling activated charcoal can be a safe way to absorb pathogens internally and topically. Activated charcoal has been treated to increase its absorptive properties, and in this DIY beauty treatment, it acts like a magnet to draw dirt and impurities from the skin.

MAKES 1 MASK

1 tablespoon bentonite clay

1 tablespoon activated charcoal powder

1 teaspoon cider vinegar

2 drops tea tree or lavender oil

Place the clay, charcoal, vinegar, and essential oil in a small bowl, along with 2 tablespoons of water. Stir well to combine. Smooth over your face, avoiding your eyes and lips. Allow to dry, then remove with warm water and a damp washcloth.

EXFOLIATING BLACK PEPPER FOOT SCRUB

The age-old practice of detoxing through cleansing your feet has been carried out by healers through the centuries. Dirty, tired, or swollen feet are thought to be associated with unhealthy lymphatic function and toxic overload. Although modern research has yet to back this up, scrubbing and massaging your feet is a smart self-care technique that can help you get rid of anxious thoughts for the simple reason that it is so relaxing-—and it can improve your circulation in the process.

MAKES ¾ CUP

½ cup coconut oil

¼ cup kosher salt

1 tablespoon coarsely ground black pepper

2 drops black pepper essential oil

Place the oil, salt, pepper, and essential oil in a small bowl. Stir well. Massage the scrub liberally over your feet and rinse with warm water. Caution when using in the tub, as the oil in the scrub may make tub surfaces slippery.

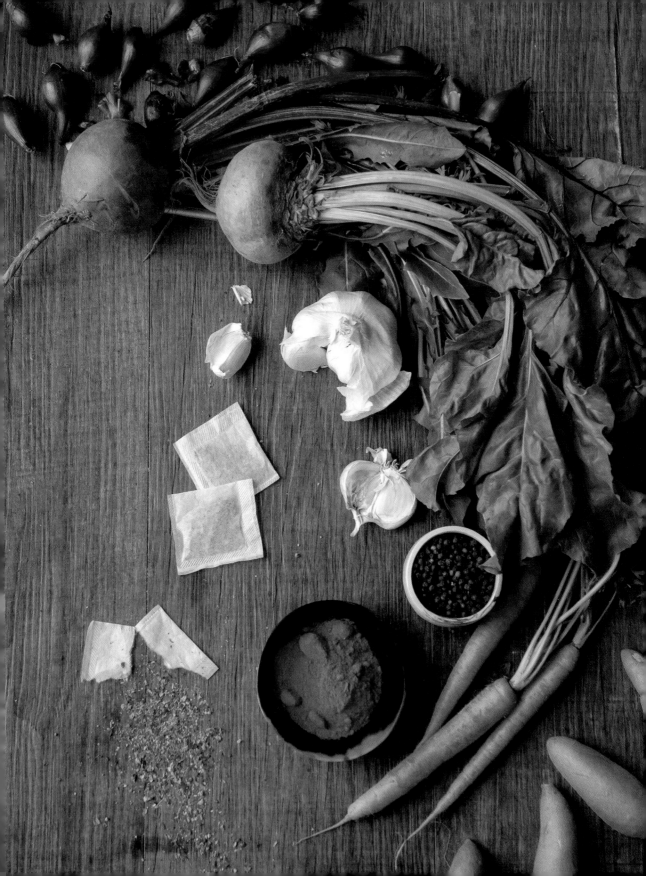

ESSENTIAL OIL CANDLE

Fire up your transformational process. Fire is the element for this chapter, and a great starting point for your own personal alchemy work; fire is a powerful way to transform material and even purify it. Nothing great can really be achieved in the chemistry lab, liquor distillery plant, or kitchen without using fire. Outside of the kitchen, lighting a candle is a soothing way to bring fire into your daily practices, for low light during meditation, as mood lighting to enjoy during a meal, or as a way to ponder the power of this feisty element.

MAKES 1 CANDLE

1 (4-ounce) candle container with lid

1 cup (8 ounces) white beeswax chips

20 drops essential oil of choice

1 wick

Remove the lid from the candle container and place the empty container on the counter.

Place the beeswax chips in the top of a double boiler over medium-low heat. Once the water starts to boil, lower the heat to low and stir the beeswax constantly until it is completely melted with no lumps, 5 to 6 minutes. The melting time will vary depending on which type of beeswax you use.

Once the wax is melted, stir in the essential oil until well incorporated. Leave the water over the lowest heat to keep it warm, since the beeswax mixture can harden quickly. Using a liquid measuring cup, carefully pour the liquid wax into your candle mold. Wrap the end of the wick around a chopstick and lower the base of it into the candle. Position the metal wick base so that it touches the bottom of the candle container with the chopstick resting across the top. Allow the candle to set for about 1 hour on the countertop to solidify, then close with the lid.

Trim the wick to 1 inch before lighting the candle.

NOTE: If you used a glass or Pyrex measuring cup when pouring the wax, fill it with hot water and use a cloth to wipe it clean. It's best to have a dedicated container for wax making.

43

Breath of Fire, or Bellows Breath

From Kundalini yoga tradition, breath of fire is a rhythmic breath with equal emphasis on the inhale and exhale to warm the body and wake up the energy. Alchemists call it the bellows breath; the bellows is the tool used to stoke the fire with air. Alchemists consider fire energy one of the greatest sources of power we have. Practicing breath of fire will help you to reinvigorate yourself and clear away pesky thoughts as you get ready for meditation. It also helps energize and oxygenate the blood, and it is a great way to shake off sleep and build stronger core muscles.

Breath of fire is practiced through the nostrils with the mouth and eyes at half-mast or closed. If you experience dizziness or lightheadedness, slow down the pace or take a small break. Beginners can start with one 30-second interval and breathe at a slower pace. As you practice breath of fire on a more regular basis, you'll build your stamina by adding more time. Avoid breath of fire if you are pregnant or menstruating. Do not do breath of fire on a full stomach or after drinking a lot of water, as fire and water don't mix.

Find a comfortable seat, cross-legged on the floor if you are flexible or seated in a chair with your legs uncrossed and feet firmly planted on the floor. Sit up as tall as you can, with a straight spine. Set a timer for 30 seconds. Lower your eyelids. With your mouth closed, take one slow breath in and out through the nose to a count of four to prep.

Next, breathe quickly in and out through the nose. Every time you breathe out, pull your abdomen in toward the spine to give push or energy to the exhale. As you release the belly, the inhale will happen naturally.

Start to shorten each breath and pick up the pace, but don't force it too much. The breathing should be loud and quick, making a puffing sound. As you breathe more quickly, the inhale and exhale will become stronger and actually sound like a bellows stoking a blazing fire. Once the timer sounds, take a break and breathe normally. You will feel a tingling, energized sensation, which is completely normal. After you become more proficient, opt for two sets of 30 seconds, or more with small breaks of calm regular breathing in between smooth, long breaths.

Meditation for Stoking the Fire and Dealing with Thoughts

Detox is important not only for the body but also for the mind. Everyone wants to have the freedom to do their best, go after their dream job, and find love, but few people realize that very often, what is standing in their way are not resources, money, or looks but, rather, negative thought patterns. What you think has so much to do with how you act and what you manifest. You can bring in fire imagery to symbolically "burn out" negative thinking.

Regular meditation stimulates the lateral prefrontal cortex (the logic center of your brain), where you can override knee-jerk emotional reactions that reinforce bad habits, such as emotional eating (see page 48) or negative self-talk. Regular meditation also keeps your medial prefrontal cortex balanced. That's the "me, myself, and I" part of the brain where you process info about your needs in relation to others, so that you have healthy feelings of empathy without being too stuck on yourself, harmonize better with others, and can enjoy richer relationships.

Fire can be a force of destruction, but it also has powers of creation and purification. This meditation invites you to visualize fire to take advantage of its cleansing properties to remove stubborn negative thoughts and beliefs. To begin this meditation, do 30 seconds or more of breath of fire (page 44) to warm up your body. Find a comfortable seat, cross-legged on the floor if you are flexible or sit in a chair with your legs uncrossed and feet firmly planted on the floor. Alternatively, you can sit on the floor with your back to a wall or piece of furniture for support. Sit up as tall as you can and still be comfortable, with a straight spine.

Begin to breathe in and out to a count of four. Imagine that you are sitting in the dark, the night sky above you, a few stars peeking through clouds as a cool breeze tingles your arms. In front of you is a large fire pit, stacked high with dry driftwood. Look into the center of the pit, focusing on the smallest, dry whitest twig in the center. Think of a handful of thoughts or habits you wish to rid yourself of. Place them near the twig or tuck them into the spaces between the driftwood. Return your attention to the center twig, breathing in and out, envisioning it in detail. Watch as the spark of your concentration lights fire to the twig. Watch as the flame grows, catching on neighboring twigs, allowing the fire to expand. Lean closer to fire, feeling the heat on your face, continuing to breathe in and out. Hear the crackling of the wood as the fire consumes it along with your unwanted thoughts. Allow yourself to be mesmerized by the bonfire you've created; as the flames lick, notice the various colors, orange, yellow with a flick of blue and green.

Healing Stone Therapy

Smoky quartz, garnet, and hematite are all healing crystals for this area. While practicing any of the meditations featured in this book, you can rest one of these crystals on your pelvis. You can also carry these crystals in your pocket during the day to feel more grounded.

Now, see the flames starting to die down, the wood beginning to smolder and smoke, and allow the cooler breeze to return. Breathe normally. Slowly open your eyes, moving your hands and feet. Gently rotate the head around to release the neck, giving your shoulders a gentle rub. Slowly rise and resume your day.

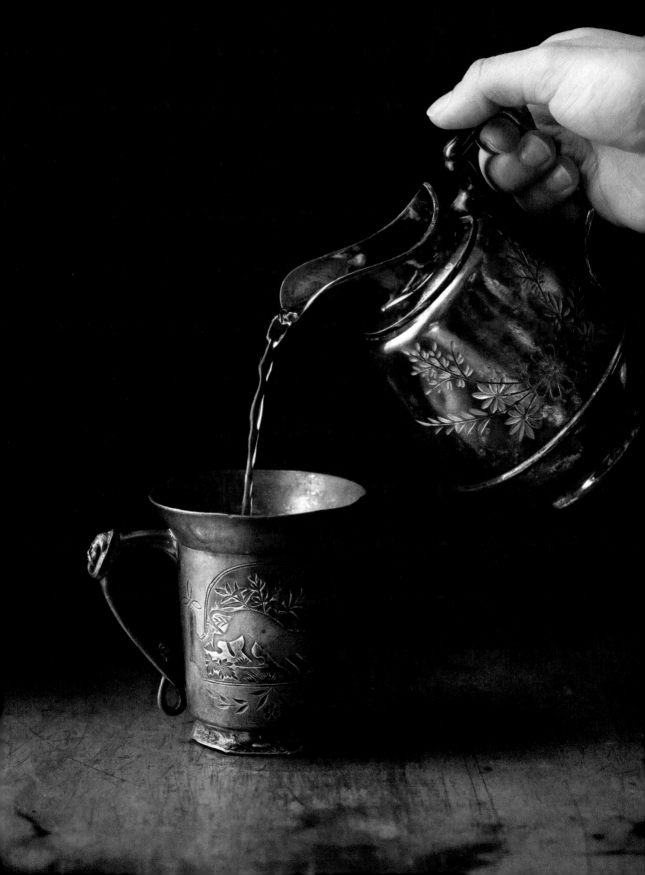

Solution

RELEASING BLOCKAGES AND
SUPPORTING THE KIDNEYS AND ADRENALS

Solution is the action or process of being dissolved in liquid. Emotion has long been associated with the element of water perhaps due to the fact that tears are triggered by strong emotions. Alchemists view crying as one of the best ways to deal with hurts and troubles from the past, as tears can dissolve and loosen "calcified" thoughts that seem to be lodged in the mind and heart. If you feel emotionally overwrought most days or are currently dealing with emotional trauma, this is a great energy center to focus on, since long-term stress can affect this area.

The recipes and therapies in this chapter correspond to the energy center surrounding the kidneys and adrenals and also the reproductive organs. The adrenals are involved in producing more than fifty hormones that drive almost every bodily function and release stress hormones such as cortisol (fight or flight) and testosterone. You may have heard of "adrenal fatigue"; the medical community is still in hot debate as to whether it is a real condition but many believe that chronic stress can overload the adrenal glands causing a host of issues throughout the body. Restoring your energy after hectic work days when you feel emotionally spent is one of the best ways to care for your adrenals. (Be cautious with caffeine since too much of it can overwork your adrenals. One safe way to give your adrenals some love is to simply decrease your caffeine intake and substitute any of the caffeine-free herbal teas in this book.) The kidneys meanwhile are involved with waste management in the body. Caring for your kidneys starts by staying properly hydrated throughout the day with water—the old wisdom of eight glasses a day is still true. Superfoods for this energy center are high in water content also providing a great way to hydrate. Sticking to a lower-sodium diet (1,500 mg a day) can also be helpful for kidney health. Since this energy center also includes the reproductive organs you'll find recipes with sweeter vegetables and fruits that have a luscious aphrodisiac-like quality along with foods traditionally linked to passion such as vanilla and spicy hot chiles.

In a chapter about emotion, I'd be remiss if I didn't also mention emotional eating. Emotional eating is the use of food as a coping mechanism. If you are an emotional eater, you have probably developed a habit of using food to self-soothe, briefly check out, or seek some relief, even when you're not hungry. Over time, it can become a very hard pattern to break. If you have ever tried to think your way out of emotional eating, you may know that it often backfires and just makes you want to eat more. However, the mind and body are deeply connected, and using body cues can be a way to deal with issues that can't be solved logically. I always recommend that people seek professional help to address emotional eating, but the following is the exercise I used to break my own cycle and it is compatible with other therapies, so I offer it here.

As soon as you have the urge to emotionally eat, notice whether part of your body has become tense. In my case, it was my stomach; I would tighten my abdomen around my navel, and then I would experience a sinking feeling and the urge to eat. Totally release that part of your body that tenses. (If you don't notice any particular sensation in your body and just take action as soon as the thought enters your head, such as jumping up from your chair to go to the fridge, then start thinking of that action as your body response or trigger for the time being. Instead of relaxing a body part in the moment, just consciously pause; if you've jumped up, sit back down.) Notice what happens to your thoughts when you relax your body. If you do move through and continue to eat, don't judge yourself; just keep up with the exercise daily. After a week, you should start to feel a slight distance from your urges. Continue the exercise until the urge subsides. Also, often the desire to eat is solved by drinking something instead, which is a good way to get those eight glasses of liquid.

Superfoods, Herbs, and Essential Oils for the Kidneys and Adrenals

BERRIES: These sweet, low-cal, fiber-rich fruits are high in water content; studies show that their antioxidant profile helps detoxify your kidneys and boost renal health.

CHERRIES: Lush cherries also deliver healing antioxidants while they hydrate. Their ruby red pigment, anthocyanin, is a protective against heart disease and other inflammatory illnesses. Cherries can carry the buildup of uric acid, which is helpful for kidney health.

GINGER: This mega anti-inflammatory root is considered to be an adaptogen because it balances as it calms. It adds a lemony kick to cooking, due to a detoxifying agents called gingerols, your new immunity partner!

PEPPERS: Peppers are high in water content and provide high levels of essential nutrients for organ health, such as vitamins A, B_6, and C.

FENNEL: In folk medicine, fennel has been used to support reproductive health. This mild, slightly sweet bulb is superhydrating and can keep water in your body longer.

CINNAMON: Superspice cinnamon has a naturally sweet taste without adding sugar; what's more, it can help balance blood sugar. It is very high in fiber and pairs well with high-water vegetables and fruits, such as peppers and watermelon.

ORANGE OR WILD ORANGE ESSENTIAL OIL: A juicy fruit with a sweet summery fragrance that can add freshness and sweetness at the same time and is used in aromatherapy to lift your mood.

SANDALWOOD ESSENTIAL OIL: The sweetest of the tree oils, this gives a woodier sweet smell and is ideal for perfuming the room and your body.

ALOE VERA: Use juicy aloe vera with foods and treatments that can soothe and balance in solution after the burn of calcination and other "fiery" alchemy work.

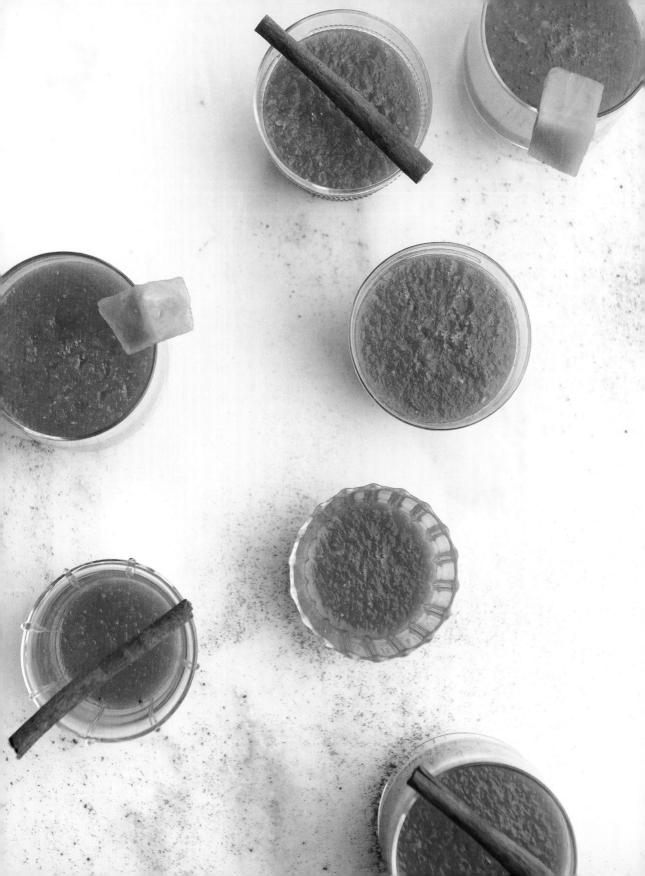

Parched after a tough workout or a day in the sun? This refreshing beverage cools as it hydrates, with vitamin C–rich red bell pepper and sweet watermelon. Goji berries add protein and loads of antioxidants in this lower-calorie drink. The hydrator can also be frozen for a highly nutritious superfood slushie.

WATERMELON
Bell Pepper Hydrator

Place the watermelon, bell pepper, goji berries, cinnamon, and ice in a blender. Blend until smooth and serve immediately.

SERVES 2

2 cups cubed watermelon

1 red bell pepper, seeded and stemmed

2 tablespoons goji berries

Pinch of ground cinnamon

4 ice cubes

---

1 cup	
94	*calories*
0 g (0 g)	*fat (sat)*
21 g	*carbs*
16 g	*sugar*
3 g	*fiber*
3 g	*protein*
23 mg	*sodium*

51

Berries spiked with ginger add tang to this creamy dessert shake. You can also use the same flavors in a healthier smoothie for breakfast: replace the ice cream with ⅔ cup of vanilla protein powder or plain Greek yogurt.

BERRY GINGER
Milk Shake

SERVES 2

2 scoops (about ½ cup) vanilla dairy or coconut ice cream

½ cup coconut milk

1 banana

1 cup raspberries

1 tablespoon chopped fresh ginger

Place the ice cream, coconut milk, banana, raspberries, and ginger in a blender. Blend on high speed for 1 minute. Divide between two glasses and serve immediately.

2½ *cups*	
294	*calories*
23 g (18 g)	*fat (sat)*
19 g	*carbs*
9 g	*sugar*
4 g	*fiber*
3 g	*protein*
18 mg	*sodium*

If you like classic chiles rellenos (stuffed chiles), you'll love this version that skips the fried crust but still brings all the roasted, smoky flavor. Search out poblano peppers, a thin-skinned low-heat chile native to Mexico, in your local specialty food market or at the farmers' market. For the sauce, look for dried ground chile peppers, such as ancho, not regular chili powder, which contains salt and other spices.

Stuffed Peppers
WITH RED ENCHILADA SAUCE

SERVES 4

To prepare the enchilada sauce, heat the butter or olive oil in a small saucepan over medium heat. Add the onion, cilantro, and garlic. Cook, stirring often, for 3 to 4 minutes, or until the onion starts to soften. Add the stock, ground chile pepper, stevia, salt, and black pepper. Stir well and cover. Cook over low heat for 45 to 50 minutes, or until the mixture is thick and the chile powder is no longer gritty.

Set the oven to BROIL. Place the poblanos on a baking sheet and roast for 4 to 5 minutes turning often, or until the skins blacken. Transfer to a bowl and cover with plastic wrap. Allow to cool. Remove and discard the skin and seeds.

Meanwhile, preheat the oven to 400°F. Fill the peppers with the refried beans and the cilantro and arrange the stuffed peppers in a 7 by 11-inch baking dish. Spoon the enchilada sauce over the stuffed peppers. Bake for 25 to 30 minutes, or until the tops of the peppers start to brown. Serve immediately.

ENCHILADA SAUCE
1 tablespoon unsalted grass-fed butter or olive oil

2 tablespoons minced red onion or shallot

2 tablespoons minced cilantro

1 garlic clove, minced

2 cups vegetable stock

½ cup mild ground chile pepper

1 teaspoon stevia or honey

½ teaspoon salt

¼ teaspoon freshly ground black pepper

4 large chiles, such as poblano or red bell peppers

1 (15-ounce) can refried beans

½ cup chopped fresh cilantro

— ◇ —
per serving
220 calories
7 g (3 g) *fat (sat)*
34 g *carbs*
4 g *sugar*
9 g *fiber*
10 g *protein*
613 mg *sodium*
— ◇ —

Bored with the same old salad? Try this spicy Latin flavor combination of chipotles and turmeric over watercress and fiber-rich black beans. If you're looking for more protein, add four boiled eggs or a half pound of cooked cubed tofu to make this salad more filling.

Watercress Salad
WITH SPICY TURMERIC GOJI BERRY DRESSING

SERVES 4

1 pound watercress

1 pound grape or cherry tomatoes, halved, or 1 orange, sectioned

1 (15-ounce) can black beans, drained, rinsed

¼ cup fresh cilantro

¼ cup goji berries

2 tablespoons olive oil

2 tablespoons cider vinegar

2 teaspoons chopped chipotle in adobo sauce

1 teaspoon ground turmeric

1 garlic clove, halved

Arrange the watercress, tomatoes, and beans in a large bowl or on a platter. Place the cilantro, goji berries, olive oil, vinegar, chipotle, turmeric, and garlic in a food processer along with ¼ cup of water. Pulse to chop until a chunky dressing forms. Drizzle over the salad and serve immediately.

per serving
176 *calories*
7 g (4 g) *fat (sat)*
30 g *carbs*
7 g *sugar*
10 g *fiber*
11 g *protein*
275 mg *sodium*

THE SUPERFOOD ALCHEMY COOKBOOK

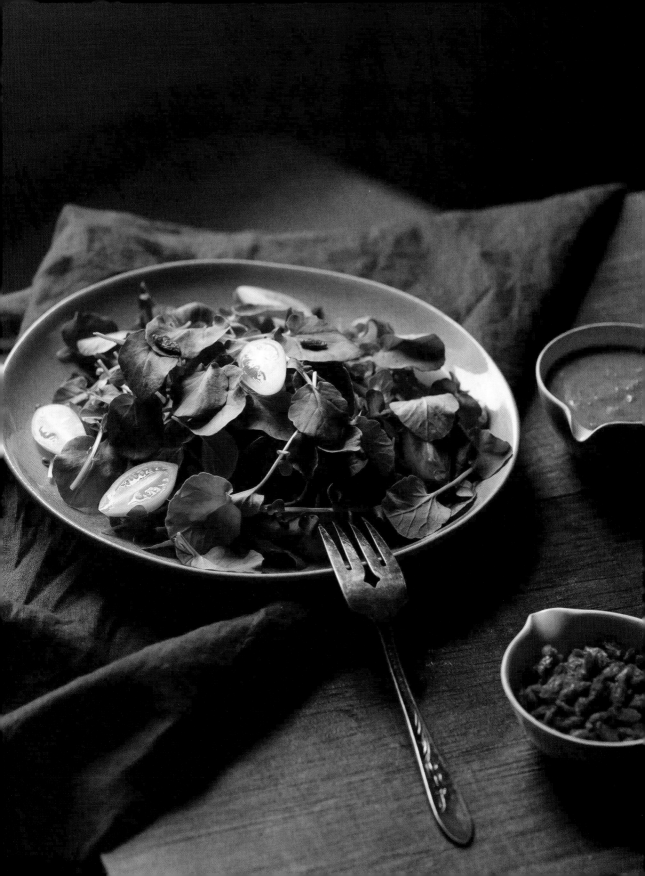

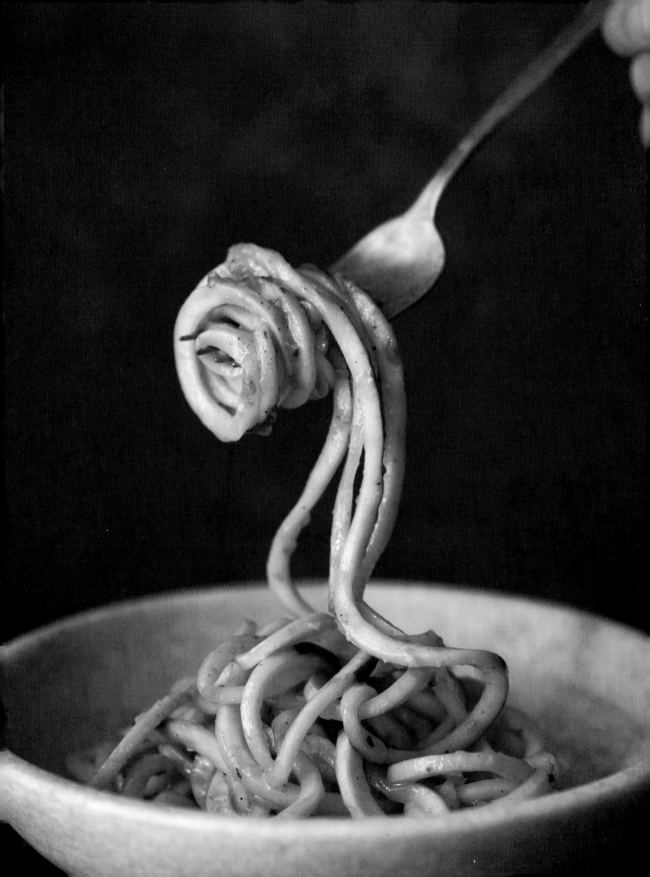

This festive dish uses two juicy superfoods for this energy center, peppers and chiles! Anyone who enjoys sweet and sour flavors will gravitate toward this dish. It's a crowd-pleaser perfect for a potluck, a starter for a romantic night in, or even a poolside nibble.

Squash Noodles
WITH ROMESCO SAUCE

SERVES 4

Preheat the oven to 450°F.

Using a spiralizer or vegetable noodle maker, process the squash into noodles.

Place the bell peppers on a baking sheet and roast, turning occasionally, for 8 to 10 minutes, or until the peppers start to blacken. Remove from the oven and let sit 5 minutes until cool enough to handle. Remove and discard the stems and seeds. Peel off and discard any blackened skin.

Place the garlic and salt in a food processor. Pulse four or five times, or until the garlic is finely chopped. Add the cilantro and almonds, pulsing again four or five times, or until finely chopped. Add the roasted peppers, tomato paste, vinegar, paprika, and cayenne. Pulse four or five times, or until a chunky sauce starts to form. Add the olive oil and pulse one or two times to blend the oil into the sauce.

Coat a large skillet with cooking spray. Heat over medium-high heat and add the vegetable noodles. Cook, tossing occasionally, for 2 to 3 minutes, or until the noodles start to soften. Turn off the heat and toss the noodles with the sauce. Serve immediately.

4 yellow squash or combination of yellow squash and zucchini (about 2 pounds)

3 red bell peppers

1 garlic clove

½ teaspoon salt

¼ cup packed fresh cilantro

¼ cup almonds

2 tablespoons tomato paste

2 tablespoons vinegar

1 teaspoon paprika

½ teaspoon cayenne or chipotle chile powder

¼ cup olive oil

Cooking spray

---
per serving
231 *calories*
19 g (3 g) *fat (sat)*
14 g *carbs*
8 g *sugar*
5 g *fiber*
5 g *protein*
320 mg *sodium*

57

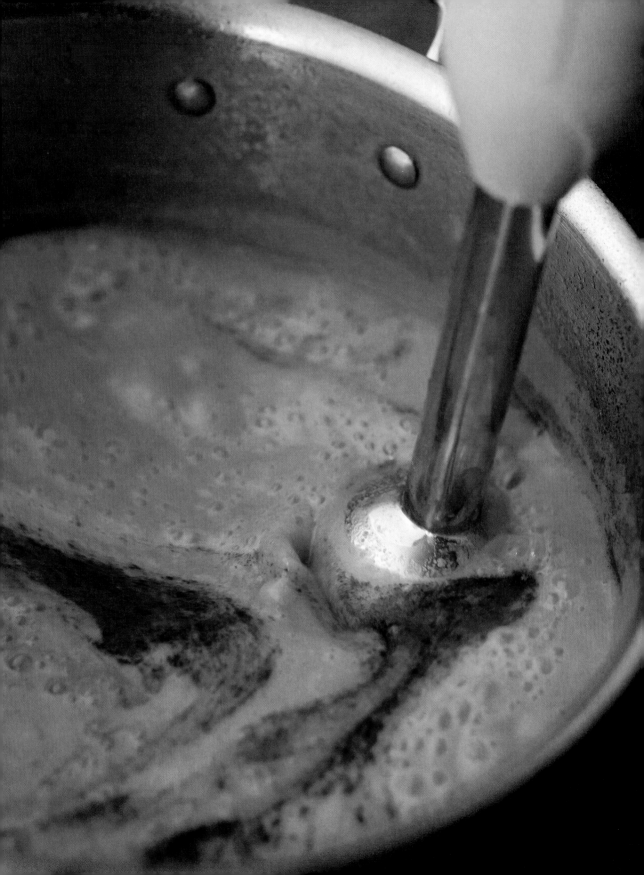

This is a delicious and comforting soup that feels like someone is giving you a big hug. Carrots are high in antioxidants, which may reduce the risk of cancer and other cardiovascular diseases. Goji berry powder is a great ingredient to have on hand but you may need to order it online; in a pinch, substitute dried cranberries.

Red Bell Pepper Carrot Soup WITH CINNAMON

Heat the oil in a large stockpot over medium heat. Add the onion, garlic, chili powder, black pepper, cinnamon, and cayenne (if using) and cook for 3 to 5 minutes. Add the carrots and stir to coat with oil. Add the stock, lower the heat to a simmer, and cover. Simmer for 40 to 45 minutes, or until the carrots are tender. Remove from the heat and stir in the chopped bell pepper. Allow to cool slightly.

Puree in a blender in batches or food processor until smooth. If the soup is too thick, add ¼ to ½ cup of water to reach your desired thickness. Garnish with the goji powder and coconut and serve.

3 tablespoons olive oil or unsalted grass-fed butter

1 small onion, finely chopped

2 garlic cloves, thinly sliced

1 teaspoon mild red chili powder or paprika

¼ teaspoon freshly ground black pepper

¼ teaspoon ground cinnamon

¼ teaspoon cayenne pepper (optional)

1 pound carrots, peeled and chopped (about 8 carrots)

1 quart vegetable stock

1 red bell pepper, seeded and chopped

4 teaspoons goji berry powder

4 teaspoons grated coconut

per serving
207 *calories*
13 g (2 g) *fat (sat)*
18 g *carbs*
9 g *sugar*
5 g *fiber*
7 g *protein*
472 mg *sodium*

You'll want to put this jam on everything! Chiles have natural capsaicin, which may be able to help your metabolic and vascular health. This condiment is a fantastic dip for veggies and really anything that needs a spicy kick.

Sweet Chile Jam

MAKES 8 SERVINGS

6 long fresh red or green chiles, stemmed and quartered

1 (2-inch-square) piece red onion

2 garlic cloves

¼ cup distilled white vinegar

Juice of 1 lime

¼ teaspoon salt

¼ cup honey

Place the chiles, onion, and garlic in a food processor and finely chop. Place in a small saucepan along with vinegar, lime juice, and salt. Cover and simmer over low heat for 10 to 15 minutes, or until the vegetables are tender and the water is evaporated. Turn off the heat and allow to cool. Once cool, stir in the honey. Transfer to an airtight container and refrigerate. Use within 1 week.

per serving
52 *calories*
0 g (0 g) *fat (sat)*
13 g *carbs*
11 g *sugar*
1 g *fiber*
1 g *protein*
77 mg *sodium*

Crepes are very thin French pancakes that have spread in popularly across the globe, no doubt because of how delicious, versatile, and crave-worthy they are. The batter is easy to whip up right in the blender, and tastes like the real deal minus the gluten.

Cherry Crepes
WITH ELDERBERRY SYRUP

Place all the ingredients, except the cooking spray, elderberry syrup, and cherries, in a blender and blend until smooth. Let sit for about 15 minutes at room temperature to thicken to the consistency of heavy cream.

Coat a small skillet with cooking spray. Heat over medium-high heat. Using a ¼-cup measure, pour the batter onto the skillet. Tilt the pan, in a circular motion, to spread the batter to coat. Cook for 3 to 4 minutes, or until the edges start to brown. Lightly spray the tops of the crepes with cooking spray, then flip. Cook for an additional 2 to 3 minutes, or until browned. Transfer to a plate and repeat with the remaining batter. Divide the crepes among six plates, drizzle with the elderberry syrup, and top with cherries.

SERVES 6

2½ cups unsweetened coconut or almond milk

2 tablespoons unsalted grass-fed butter, melted, or olive oil

2 teaspoons honey, agave nectar, or stevia

1 cup gluten-free multipurpose flour

¼ cup ground flax meal

½ teaspoon ground ginger

½ teaspoon gluten-free baking powder

½ teaspoon pure vanilla extract

Cooking spray

6 tablespoons elderberry syrup

2 cups fresh or frozen pitted cherries (thaw if frozen)

◇
---

per serving
156 *calories*
5 g (3 g) *fat (sat)*
22 g *carbs*
5 g *sugar*
0 g *fiber*
3 g *protein*
34 mg *sodium*

◇

Tomatoes are a great source of lycopene, which may help fight cancer-causing free radicals. When combined with refreshingly sweet papaya, you have a crave-worthy duo. Feel free to add any other fragrant herbs you have on hand. A taste of the tropics awaits your palate!

TOMATO PAPAYA
Black Pepper Soup

SERVES 4

1 pound heirloom or plum tomatoes

2 tablespoons olive oil

2 teaspoons fresh thyme or rosemary leaves, chopped

½ teaspoon salt

1 teaspoon freshly ground black pepper

1 (2-pound) papaya

2 cups vegetable stock

½ teaspoon ground cayenne pepper (optional)

½ cup fresh basil leaves

Preheat the oven or a toaster oven to 450°F. Quarter the tomatoes and place them on a baking sheet, skin side down. Drizzle the tops of the tomatoes with the olive oil. Sprinkle with the thyme or rosemary, salt, and ½ teaspoon of the black pepper. Bake for 25 to 30 minutes, or until the tomatoes start to brown. Remove from the oven and allow the tomatoes to cool on the baking sheet for 15 to 20 minutes.

While the tomatoes are cooling, peel the skin from the papaya with a potato peeler. Cut the papaya in half and scoop out the dark seeds, discarding them. Cut the papaya halves into quarters.

Transfer the papaya to a blender along with the roasted tomatoes and any juice from the baking sheet. Add the stock and blend until smooth. Divide among four bowls and garnish with the remaining ½ teaspoon of black pepper, the cayenne (if using), and the basil leaves. Serve immediately.

per serving	
123	*calories*
8 g (1 g)	*fat (sat)*
14 g	*carbs*
9 g	*sugar*
3 g	*fiber*
2 g	*protein*
733 mg	*sodium*

THE SUPERFOOD ALCHEMY COOKBOOK

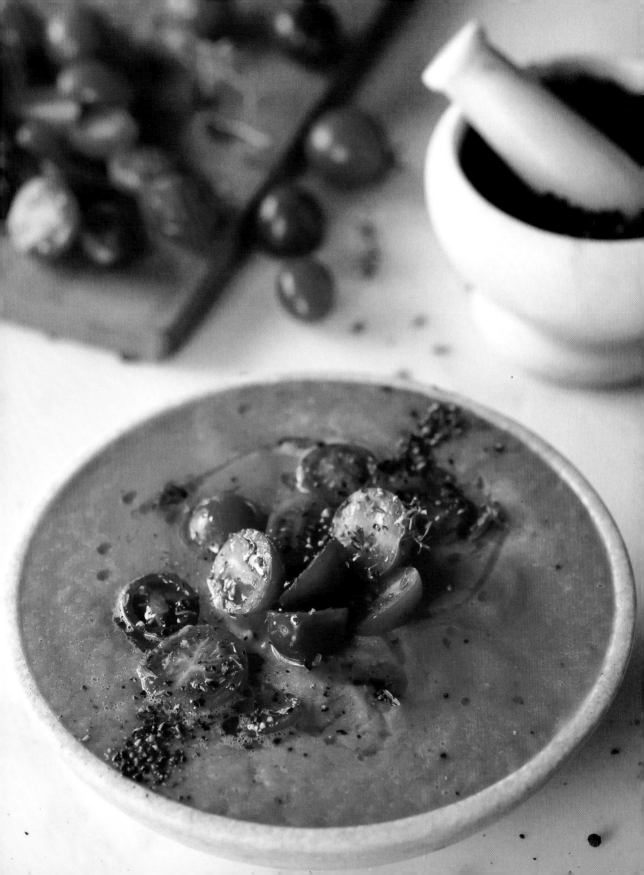

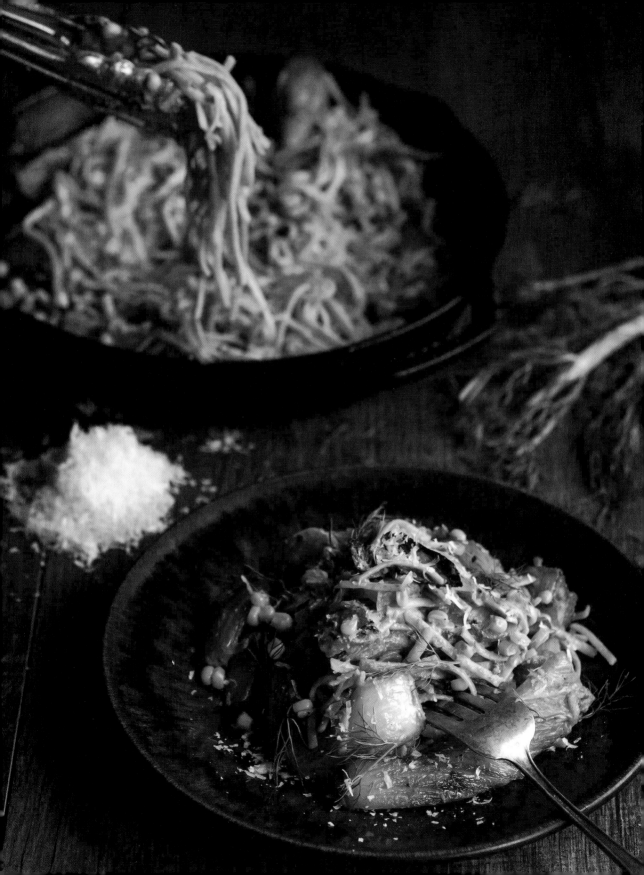

Charred fennel bulb is a beloved, licorice-scented vegetable dish that has passed the test of time, trends, and generations. Here we combine its sweet, luxurious taste with a gluten-free pasta and shaved Parmesan. If you're avoiding traditional pasta for any reason, you could also try this with yellow squash noodles. For those who are watching their sodium intake (important for kidney health!), check the ingredients on your pasta before you buy; some brands are salt-free but others do contain salt.

CHARRED FENNEL SAMBUCA
Corn Pasta

SERVES 6

Cook the pasta according to the package instructions, then drain, reserving ½ cup of the cooking liquid, and set aside.

Heat the olive oil in a large skillet, preferably cast iron, over medium heat. Add the fennel, salt, and pepper. Cook for 20 to 25 minutes, or until the fennel is very soft and starts to char around the edges, turning occasionally. Add the garlic and cook for 1 minute more, or until the garlic starts to brown. Carefully add the sambuca (if using) and cook for 2 to 3 minutes more, or until most of the liquid evaporates. Add the corn, Parmesan or nutritional yeast, cream, reserved pasta cooking water, and pasta. Toss well.

12 ounces gluten-free pasta, such as corn or quinoa

3 tablespoons olive oil

2 fennel bulbs, thinly sliced

¾ teaspoon salt

½ teaspoon freshly ground black pepper

4 garlic cloves, thinly sliced

2 tablespoons tomato paste

¼ cup sambuca or other licorice-flavored liqueur (optional)

2 cups fresh or frozen corn kernels (thaw if frozen)

1 cup grated Parmesan cheese, or ¼ cup nutritional yeast

½ cup heavy cream or coconut cream

---
per serving
473 *calories*
20 g (8 g) *fat (sat)*
64 g *carbs*
4 g *sugar*
8 g *fiber*
13 g *protein*
598 mg *sodium*

65

SOLUTION

This Moroccan spin on curry brings the sweet, floral tastes of almonds and apricots that contrast with the spicy heat of Thai curry paste. Pair this dish with the Harissa-Spiced Eggplant (page 93) to create an exotic dining experience your guests will savor.

Thai Red Bell Pepper Curry
WITH ALMONDS AND APRICOT

SERVES 4

½ cup uncooked short-grain brown rice or jasmine rice

Cooking spray

1 tablespoon olive oil

4 red bell peppers, seeded and chopped

2 fennel bulbs, thinly sliced

1 onion, peeled and diced

½ teaspoon salt

1 tablespoon curry powder or red curry paste

1 (15-ounce) can coconut milk

¼ cup dried apricots, minced

¼ cup slivered almonds

Cook the rice according to the package instructions and set aside. Coat a large skillet with cooking spray, place over medium heat, and heat the olive oil in the skillet. Add the bell peppers, fennel, onion, and salt and cook for 4 to 5 minutes, or until the vegetables start to soften. Add the curry powder and cook for an additional minute, stirring often to bring out the flavor in the spices.

Reduce the heat to low and add the coconut milk. Cover and cook for 5 to 7 minutes, or until the fennel is tender and a thick sauce forms. Sprinkle the curry mixture and rice with the almonds and apricots. Serve the curry immediately over the rice or with the rice on the side.

2 cups
456 calories
26 g (20 g) fat (sat)
26 g carbs
14 g sugar
9 g fiber
10 g protein
379 mg sodium

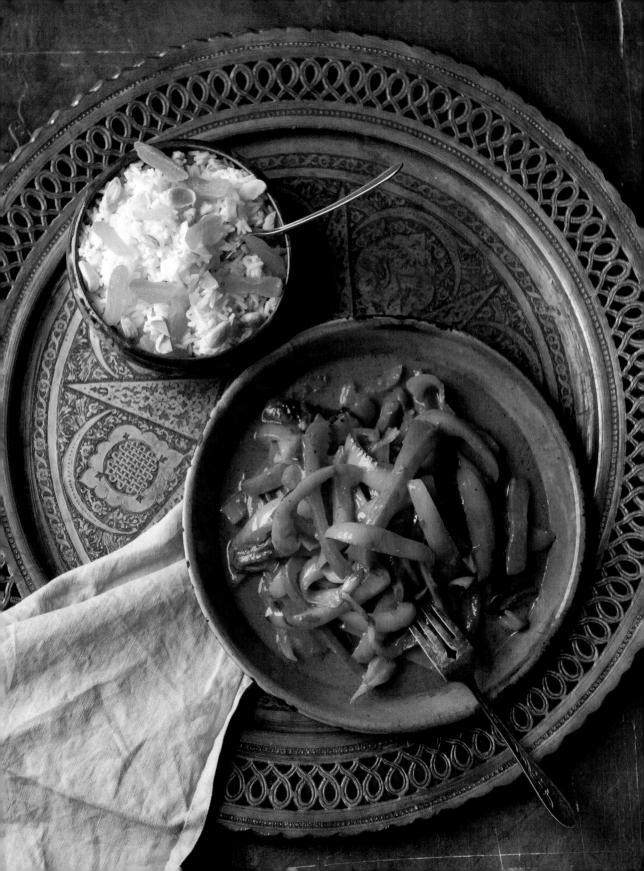

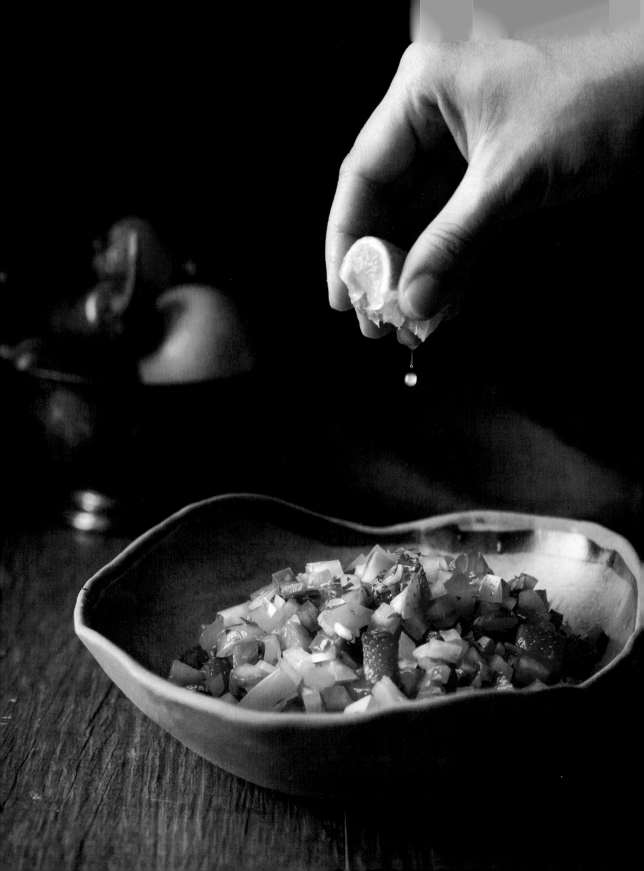

Want a novel way to impress your health-conscious guests? Try serving up this spin on traditional salsa and chips at your next dinner party. Taro is packed with vitamins A and C and contains phenolic compounds that calm inflammation while you munch.

Jalapeño Strawberry Salsa
WITH ROOT CHIPS

SERVES 4

Place the strawberries, jalapeños, cilantro, lime zest and juice, onion, bell pepper, and salt in a bowl and mix to thoroughly combine. Let sit for 5 minutes to allow the flavors to meld.

Serve with the taro root chips for dipping.

1 quart strawberries, hulled and diced

2 jalapeño peppers, minced and optionally seeded

¼ cup packed fresh cilantro leaves, minced

Zest and juice of 1 lime

2 tablespoons minced red onion

½ red bell pepper, seeded and minced

½ teaspoon salt

1 (5-ounce) package taro root chips

per serving

154	*calories*
29 g (0 g)	*fat (sat)*
29 g	*carbs*
10 g	*sugar*
5 g	*fiber*
2 g	*protein*
421 mg	*sodium*

69

This lovely, ladylike sorbet brings the delicate flavors of vanilla and cinnamon to the nutty smoothness of coconut cream and peanut butter. Ice-cream makers are inexpensive and easy to use, and allow you to make ice creams for every season. Making your sweets has triple benefits: less sugar, more healing foods, and a chance to spoil yourself without guilt.

VANILLA
Cinnamon Sorbet

SERVES 4

1 (15-ounce) can coconut milk

¼ cup honey or agave nectar, or 2 tablespoons stevia

2 tablespoons peanut butter

1 tablespoon pure vanilla extract

1 teaspoon ground cinnamon

Put all the ingredients plus 1 cup of water in a blender and blend until smooth. Transfer to an ice-cream maker and process according to the manufacturer's instructions.

per serving
330 *calories*
27 g (21 g) *fat (sat)*
23 g *carbs*
18 g *sugar*
1 g *fiber*
4 g *protein*
53 mg *sodium*

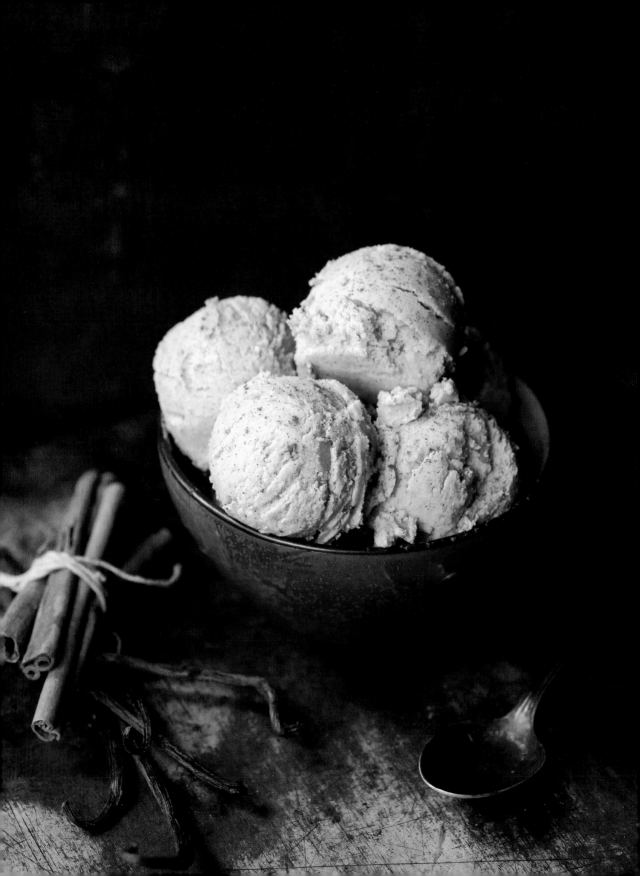

Essential Oil Preparations and Rituals for Solution

ALOE VERA ICE CUBES

Have these on hand to soothe a sunburn or remedy puffy eyes. For gentler applications, wrap the aloe vera ice cubes in a clean dish towel or washcloth and apply as a compress. You can use fresh gel from the plant or simply buy the gel, easily found online, to have on hand for multiple uses.

MAKES 16 ICE CUBES

1 cup aloe vera gel

Place the aloe vera gel in a large measuring cup along with 1 cup of cold water. Gently whisk to combine. Pour into an empty ice cube tray. Freeze for at least 1 hour before using.

SUGAR BODY SCRUB

This "sweet" scrub will soften your skin with its gritty crystals. Use this scrub for your body, avoiding you face. Since it contains oil, be careful to clean your tub as residue can make for slippery surfaces.

MAKES 1/3 CUP

4 tablespoons coconut sugar

2 tablespoons coconut oil

1 tablespoon honey

6 drops orange essential oil

6 drops calendula or lavender essential oil

Place the coconut sugar, oil, honey, and essential oils in a small bowl and stir well. Use liberally over arms and legs, rinsing with warm water.

ALOE VERA FACE SCRUB

Drinking aloe vera juice is super soothing for your digestion since it contains a special gel that can help tissues heal, but it's equally soothing when used on your face. Enjoy this easy scrub that exfoliates and soothes at the same time.

MAKES 1 TREATMENT

1 teaspoon aloe vera gel

1 teaspoon coconut sugar

1 drop geranium or rose essential oil

Place the aloe vera gel, sugar, and essential oil in a small bowl. Wet a cotton swab with water and dip in the scrub. Gently scrub your face, continuing to dip the cotton into the sugar scrub as needed. Rinse your face with cold water and dry.

ALOE VERA FACE SPRAY

Atomizers and face misters are an amazing (expensive) way to give your face a little hydration during a busy day. Making your own is not only more economical but also gives you the option of working with different scents.

MAKES ¾ CUP

2 tablespoons aloe vera gel

1 tablespoon witch hazel

1 drop lavender oil

1 drop rose or frankincense essential oil

½ cup distilled or filtered cold water

Place the aloe vera gel, witch hazel, and essential oil along with the water in a small bowl and gently whisk to combine. Transfer to a spray bottle and spritz one to two times over you face, with closed eyes. Store in a cool cabinet or refrigerate during hotter days for a cooling surprise.

ORANGE CALENDULA BUBBLE BATH

Immersing yourself in water can be a powerful ritual for healing, and hydrotherapy can help bring balance to your body and mind. Hot and cold temperatures, either used as compresses or in immersion baths, helps encourage the circulation of blood and lymphatic fluids in the body, directing fluids to where they are needed and flushing them out of areas that may be congested or inflamed. And water can help you connect to your emotions. So, if you haven't indulged in a bubble bath lately, know they're good for more than relaxation! Egg may seem like a strange addition to the mix, but it provides big lovely bubbles that you can't normally get from castile soap. If you are concerned about salmonella, clean the eggshell before you crack it, since pathogens cling to the shell and don't penetrate. This bubble bath is a great addition to the water meditation that follows.

MAKES ENOUGH FOR 2 BUBBLE BATHS

½ cup liquid castile soap

¼ cup honey

1 egg white (optional)

4 drops orange essential oil

2 drops calendula essential oil

Place the soap, honey, egg white (if using), and essential oils in a medium-size bowl. Gently stir to combine. Store in a large mason jar for to 1 week, refrigerated. Use ½ cup per bath.

Water Meditation to Move Through Emotion

Alchemists and psychologists alike believe emotions are triggered by thoughts, memories, or even stories we construct around painful or happy situations, which we continue to foster and engage with. The first operation in alchemy, calcination, uses fire to "burn up" negative thoughts (see page 44). However, what if you are still stuck on a thought or feeling that you can't seem to let go of? Look to the principles of this operation, solution, to dissolve emotions by releasing them (much like releasing hurt by crying), so that strong feelings do not cause continuous stress on your body.

Healing Stone Therapy
Carnelian, orange calcite, and hessonite garnet are all healing crystals for this area. While practicing any of the meditations featured in this book, you can rest one of these crystals a few inches below your belly button. Add them to your bath, while you bathe, to boost this energy center.

As you approach this meditation practice, try to ignore or release any feelings of competitiveness or self-judgment. Instead, throughout your meditative practice, maintain an openness to what may happen, as if you are watching an interesting movie or a marvelous dance. One of the goals of mediation is to simply witness what is happening in the mind.

Your mantra for this meditation is "just let go." Imagine that are you releasing the gates of a dam, allowing the water to pour out and flow away as you do this mediation.

Emotions behave like water, and when you understand the nature of emotions better, they are far easier to cope with. Emotions, like water, ebb and flow; they can rush in like a wave or pound the sidewalks as a furious fall rain. Emotions can also be like the weather, ever changing and highly influenced by your thoughts.

Taking a bath is one of the most instantly relaxing rituals that also cleanses your body in the process. Try this mediation paired with the Orange Calendula Bubble Bath (page 73). To begin, draw a warm bath, one that's not too hot. Add your bubble bath, if using. Enter the bath and relax, taking several slow breaths in and out, calming you thoughts as you focus your eyes on the water. Call up three memories of when you were sad: one when you were heartbroken or shocked, one when you had a fierce fight with a loved one, and one when someone disappointed you. Consider how water or rainy weather relates to each feeling: perhaps you see the feelings as a tsunami, or a chilly thunderstorm? Again, avoid any impulse to judge yourself as you recall these situations; simply observe and allow the feelings and the images to wash over you.

Now, think of three joyful incidents: perhaps one when you were passionately in love, one when you experienced family connection (or even connection with your pet), and one when a playful child made you laugh. How does water relate to these? Maybe the passion calls to mind a luscious waterfall in the tropics, whereas the family memory is like a calm lake with birds flying past at dawn on a summer day. How would you describe the playful child memory, perhaps a bird splashing in a bird bath?

Take notice of how you described the two separate groupings of experiences from sad to joyful. Where did the water scenarios take place? Were they all in the same place or did they take place at special locales? When you finish your bath, jot it down. Also take note of the transition from sad thoughts to happen ones. Did you notice that just by using your thoughts, you create your own emotional experiences? Remember, you can reuse ideas and techniques from these meditations in other situations any time you need them—this meditation takes you from sad thoughts to happy thoughts, and even being intention-al about shifting your focus can leave you with improved feelings.

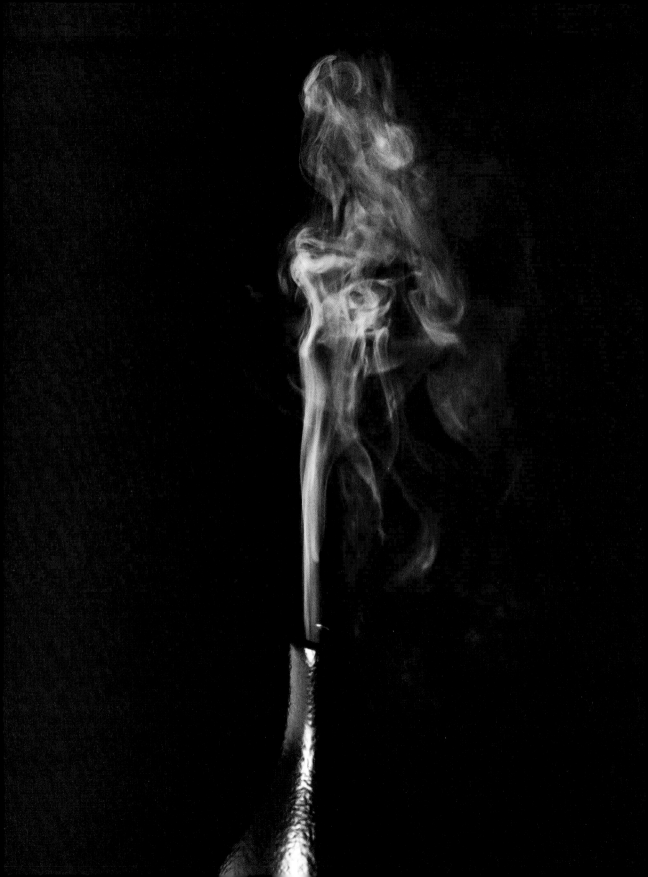

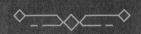
Separation

PROMOTING DIGESTION AND SUPPORTING THE GUT

Separation in alchemy signifies *"sifting through matter."*

Are you game for a career change and ready to follow your dream? Or perhaps you're ready to shrug off some old identity or break a lingering habit. You may be realizing that messages you received from your family or from society at large have limited you, and now it's time to just be yourself. Separation in alchemy signifies "sifting through matter" to keep the worthy items and discard the nonbeneficial parts, releasing criticism, shame, and judgment placed on you by others. Alchemists associate the element of air with this operation, and getting a "fresh breath of air" to center yourself. In many spiritual traditions, the area surrounding the gut is the center of confidence. Asserting your will while maintaining healthy boundaries is all a part of separation, so the tools and rituals in this chapter center on building the confidence and inner strength to do this important work.

Biologically, this energy center houses the microbiome, the jungle of organisms in your small and large intestines. Thousands of different species of microbiota *separate* particles of food with their digestive enzymes to create essential nutrients that your body needs to prevent disease, build muscle mass, and even communicate with your brain. Now that we know all about the microbiome, even the idea of "gut instinct" can be explained scientifically. Your gut actually contains 100 million neurons that it uses to communicate with

bacteria, as well as with your nervous system and brain—this is why some are starting to refer to the gut as a "second brain." When you have that notorious "pit of your stomach" feeling, it's not just the bad takeout you had last night—your nervous system is deeply linked to neurons in your gut that fire off information to signal when something isn't quite right. This form of communication is more a primitive form of thinking, not the conscious reasoning that the brain does. But the gut can quickly trigger vague feelings, impressions, and even feelings of panic or anxiety. Consider good gut bugs as "invisible alchemists" who create serotonin, a neurotransmitter that calms appetite while improving digestion. The better you treat (and feed) your gut bugs, giving them high-quality superfoods that you'll find throughout this book, the better you'll be able to react to stress. Gastroenterologists who specialize in healing the gut have a formula of "remove, replace, reinoculate, and repair." Step one is to remove highly processed sugars, gluten, and highly processed white carbs that harm the microbiome. The recipes in this chapter aim to move on to step two, to replace, by swapping out the bad and replacing them with superfoods and healing herbs that gut bugs flourish on so that plant-based eating becomes part of your life. You will also find foods that reinoculate in Chapter 5, Fermentation (page 145).

Superfoods, Herbs, and Essential Oils for the Gut

APPLES: Apples, especially the skins, are high in quercetin, a flavonoid that is protective for neural cells, helping them dispel toxins. Rich in both pectin and fiber, apples feed the microbiome and make for smoother cruising on the gut-brain highway.

AVOCADOS: These fatty fruits offer loads of fiber (a whopping 13 grams in one, which is half your daily needs). Avocados are also high in monounsaturated fatty acids (MUFA) and vitamin E, which work as antioxidants to help repair the lining of your gut while reducing hunger.

MINT AND PEPPERMINT OIL: Mint may seem like a run-of-the-mill garnish herb, but it's a helpful medicinal plant for your digestion. Mint is used widely by gastroenterologists since it contains a terpene, l-menthol, which works as a pain reducer while it calms inflammation, ideal for patients suffering from irritable bowel syndrome (IBS) and other painful digestive issues. Both mint and peppermint oil contain antimicrobial compounds that can help control harmful gut bacteria.

GOJI BERRIES: Also known as wolf berries, these high-protein, high-fiber adaptogenic berries grow on rocky crags in the Himalayas and weather some of the toughest conditions, producing antioxidants as protection again the harsh climate. They help calm inflammation in the intestines.

OREGANO AND OREGANO OIL: This herb contains the active compound carvacrol, studied as therapy against various bacterial and fungal infections. Traditionally, oregano is used to balance gut health, and in several studies, it has been found to lessen the effects of food-borne pathogens, such as the *E. coli* bacteria. Oregano oil can be used as a quick fix for cranky digestion and is prescribed by gastroenterologists to treat *Candida* overgrowth by adding the oil to drops of water (see page 107). Just check to be sure you have the food-grade variety of oil.

TULSI: Also called "holy basil," this adaptogen is from the same family as culinary basil. Used traditionally in Ayurvedic medicine, it is considered the "queen of healing" by homeopathic doctors in India. It is being studied as a potential therapy for cancer, diabetes, and microbial and fungal infections, including those in the gut, due to its active compound eugenol.

CARDAMOM AND CARDAMOM OIL: Like the spice, cardamom essential oil is a digestion soother. It can stimulate bowel flow and ease intestinal contractions when paired with proper hydration. Scent-wise, cardamom has a peppery fresh kick mixed with a spicy, nutmeg-like earthlines. Cardamom, the signature spice that gives chai tea its main yum factor, is a super soother for your gut.

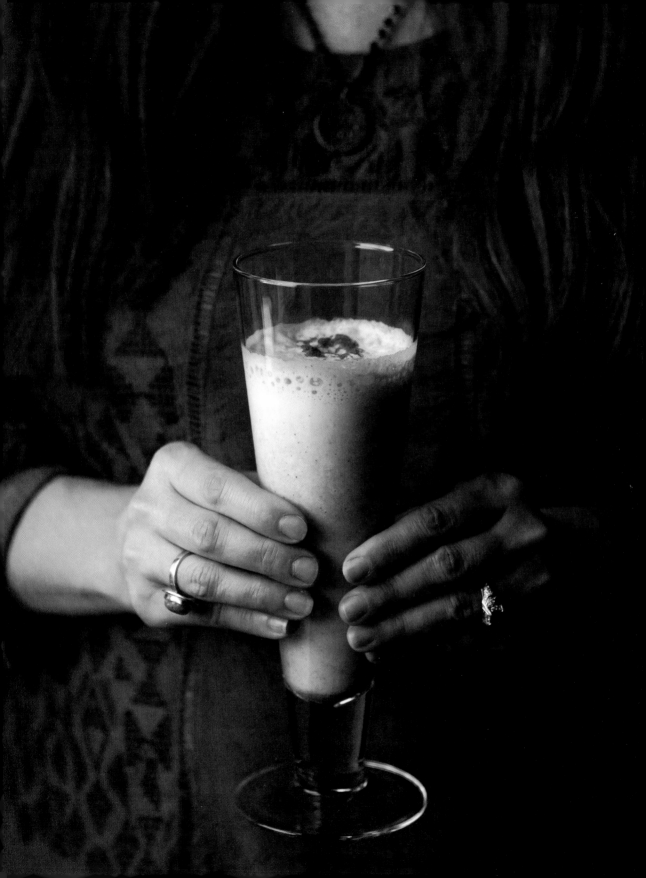

Starting your day with fiber-rich foods means less hunger pangs and snacking throughout the day, since fiber helps balance blood sugar while efficiently feeding your gut bugs. Such spices as cinnamon and cardamom add the comforting aromas along with additional antioxidants.

SPICED APPLE
Tulsi Tea Smoothie

Place all the ingredients in a blender and blend until smooth. Divide between two glasses and serve garnished with an additional sprinkle of cinnamon, if you like.

NOTE: To brew the tea, pour 1 cup of boiling water over one tulsi tea bag or 1 teaspoon of dried tulsi in an infuser. Allow to steep for at least 5 minutes, then remove the tulsi. Allow the tea to cool completely before using in this recipe.

SERVES 2

2 medium-size apples, unpeeled but cored

1 cup brewed tulsi tea

⅔ cup vanilla protein powder or plain Greek yogurt

½ cup coconut milk

¼ cup walnuts or hemp seeds

½ teaspoon almond or pure vanilla extract

½ teaspoon ground cinnamon, plus more for garnish (optional)

½ teaspoon ground cardamom

1 teaspoon stevia (optional)

8 ice cubes

2½ cups
313 *calories*
12 g (2 g) *fat (sat)*
35 g *carbs*
22 g *sugar*
9 g *fiber*
22 g *protein*
93 mg *sodium*

Serve up this superfood salad, loaded with apples and refreshing mint, at your next barbecue or cookout. Apples are rich in fiber, which boosts gut health. If you can't find goji berries, you can substitute dried cherries or cranberries, though gojis are widely available online and add an adaptogenic kick to this recipe.

CREAMY APPLE CELERY
Goji Berry Salad

SERVES 6

½ cup mayonnaise
or vegan mayonnaise

½ cup plain unsweetened
whole milk or coconut yogurt

½ cup fresh mint leaves,
chopped

½ teaspoon Dijon mustard

1 tablespoon cider vinegar

¼ teaspoon salt

¼ teaspoon ground cardamom

¼ teaspoon freshly ground
black pepper

4 apples, cored and cubed

4 celery stalks, peeled,
trimmed, and thinly sliced

¼ cup dried goji berries

Place the mayonnaise, yogurt, mint, mustard, vinegar, salt, cardamom, and pepper in a large bowl. Whisk to combine. Add the apples and celery and toss to evenly coat. Garnish with the goji berries and cover. Refrigerate for at least 1 hour before serving.

1 cup	
223	calories
14 g (3 g)	fat (sat)
23 g	carbs
1 g	sugar
4 g	fiber
2 g	protein
260 mg	sodium

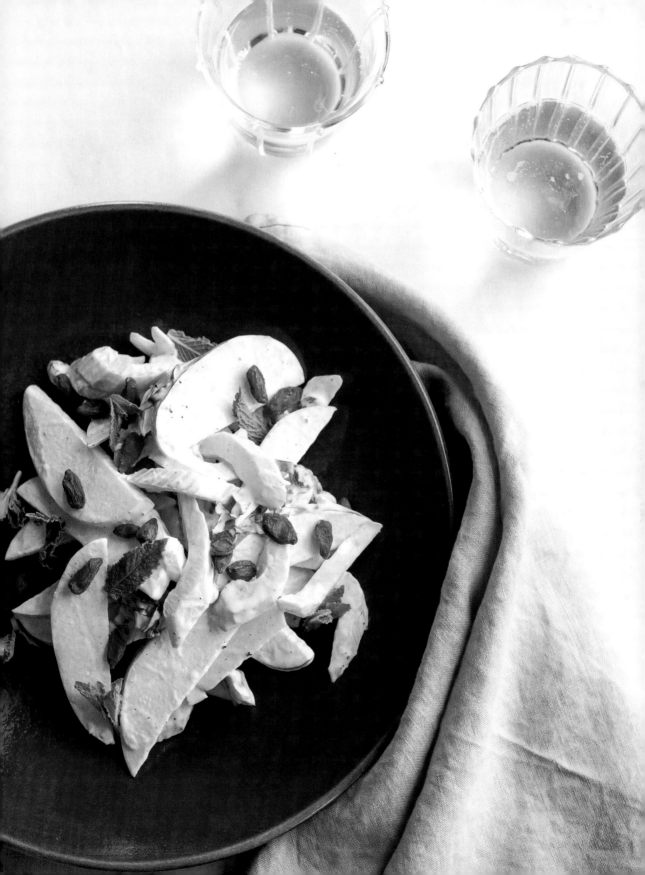

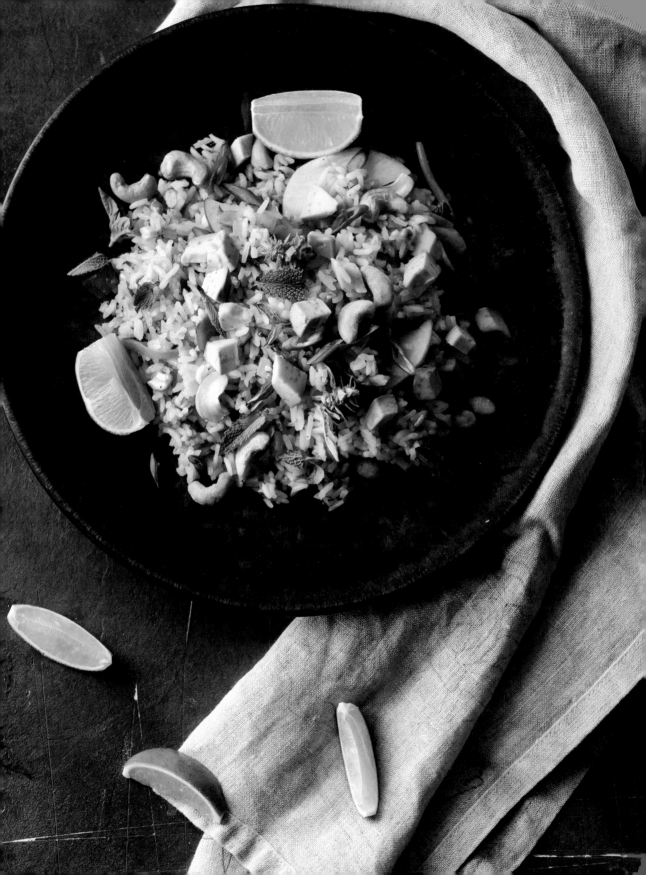

Out of all the grains, rice is the best tolerated by people with allergies and is naturally gluten-free—two pluses for gut health. Rice that is cooked and then cooled to room temperature is considered to be one of the special resistant starches, like the kind you'll find in root vegetables, which make the best food for your good gut bugs. The miso brings in additional probiotics. This luscious fried rice is topped with cooling, fiber-rich avocado and crisp sliced apple.

Avocado Fried Rice
WITH MINT AND CHILES

Cook the rice for 4 minutes less than the package instructions specify and set aside to cool to room temperature. Heat the oil in a large skillet over medium heat. Add the carrot, onion, and garlic. Cook, stirring often, for 4 to 5 minutes, or until the vegetables start to soften. Push the vegetables aside and add the rice. Cook for 1 minute, stirring the vegetables into the rice.

Lower the heat to low and add the tamari, miso paste, tomato, basil, and mint. Toss well to combine. Add the tofu and apple, toss again, and transfer to a platter. Top with the avocado and scallions. Serve the fried rice hot and squeeze the lime wedges over as desired.

SERVES 4

1 cup uncooked rice, such as short-grain or risotto

2 tablespoons olive or sesame oil

1 large carrot, peeled and diced small or julienned

½ onion, minced

2 garlic cloves, minced

1 to 2 tablespoons low-sodium tamari

2 tablespoons white or yellow miso paste

1 tomato, chopped

½ cup fresh regular or Thai basil leaves, thinly sliced

½ cup fresh mint leaves, thinly sliced

4 ounces tofu, patted dry and cut in ½-inch dice, or 1 cup cashews

1 apple, cored and thinly sliced

2 avocados, pitted, peeled, and cubed

4 scallions, thinly sliced

2 limes, cut into wedges

per serving with 1 tbsp. tamari
307 *calories*
9 g (1 g) *fat (sat)*
51 g *carbs*
8 g *sugar*
6 g *fiber*
8 g *protein*
689 mg *sodium*

85

Goji berries are a superfood whose intense pink pigment signals a high load of antioxidants, as well as vitamins A, B_2, and C, iron, and selenium. Their sweet, chewy texture make them a great addition to this warm, savory combo of caramelized apples and onions.

GOJI CARAMELIZED CINNAMON
Apples and Onions

SERVES 4

3 tablespoons olive oil

4 firm apples, preferably Fuji, Gala, or Pink Lady, cored and sliced

2 white or yellow onions, sliced

½ teaspoon ground cinnamon

½ teaspoon salt

¼ teaspoon freshly ground black pepper

2 tablespoons dried goji berries

Heat 1½ teaspoons of the oil in a large, cast-iron skillet over medium-low heat. Add the apples and onions and cook, stirring occasionally, for 5 to 8 minutes, or until slightly softened and starting to brown. Transfer the mixture to a platter or bowl. Toss with the cinnamon, salt, pepper, and remaining 1½ teaspoons of olive oil. Scatter the goji berries on top. Serve warm.

per serving
219 *calories*
10 g (1 g) *fat (sat)*
33 g *carbs*
23 g *sugar*
6 g *fiber*
2 g *protein*
304 mg *sodium*

THE SUPERFOOD ALCHEMY COOKBOOK

Full of delicious herbs and refreshing yogurt, this chilled soup is a play on the flavors of Mediterranean tzatziki sauce. Cucumbers are a great source of phytonutrients, which have antioxidant and anti-inflammatory properties. Feel free to play around with this recipe and add any fresh herbs you have on hand.

COOLING
Cucumber Soup

SERVES 4

Place cucumbers, yogurt, stock, lemon juice, cilantro, basil, tamari, garlic salt, and pepper in a blender and process until smooth. Divide among four bowls. Drizzle each with olive oil and top with a quarter of the avocado. Serve immediately.

2 cucumbers, halved and seeded

1 cup whole Greek or coconut yogurt

½ cup vegetable stock

2 tablespoons freshly squeezed lemon juice (from ½ lemon)

¼ cup fresh cilantro leaves

2 tablespoons chopped fresh basil

1 tablespoon gluten-free tamari

½ teaspoon garlic salt

⅛ teaspoon freshly ground black pepper

4 teaspoons olive oil

1 avocado, pitted, peeled, and thinly sliced

1 cup
179 calories
13 g (3 g) fat (sat)
12 g carbs
5 g sugar
3 g fiber
7 g protein
243 mg sodium

The key to eating well is making things you love in a healthier, more nutritious way. If you love those crisp iceberg wedge salads, don't scrap them completely; make this more nutrient-dense swap. Eating salad on a regular basis is a great practice for your gut, since certain greens contain detoxifying compounds, such as vitamin A, that can repair damaged gut tissues.

Romaine Lettuce Wedges
WITH GREEK DRESSING

SERVES 4

1 pound romaine lettuce heads (about 3 heads)

¼ cup olive oil

¼ cup red wine or cider vinegar

1 garlic clove, minced

2 teaspoons dried oregano

½ teaspoon salt

¼ teaspoon freshly ground black pepper

1 teaspoon honey or stevia

1 pound tomatoes, diced

1 cucumber, diced

1 red bell pepper, seeded and sliced

1 cup cubed feta or firm tofu

2 tablespoons hemp or chia seeds (optional)

Trim the ends of the lettuce heads. Fill two large bowls with lukewarm water and add the lettuce heads. Soak for 10 minutes, then remove from the water and place in a colander to drain for 5 minutes. Wrap in paper towels or tea towels and refrigerate at least 1 hour, or until crisp.

Place the olive oil, vinegar, garlic, oregano, salt, black pepper, and honey or stevia in a bowl and whisk well to combine. Arrange the lettuce, tomato, cucumber, red bell pepper, and feta or tofu in a large bowl or on a large platter. Drizzle with the dressing and sprinkle with hemp or chia seeds (if using). Serve immediately.

per serving
315 *calories*
24 g (8 g) *fat (sat)*
15 g *carbs*
9 g *sugar*
3 g *fiber*
11 g *protein*
938 mg *sodium*

THE SUPERFOOD ALCHEMY COOKBOOK

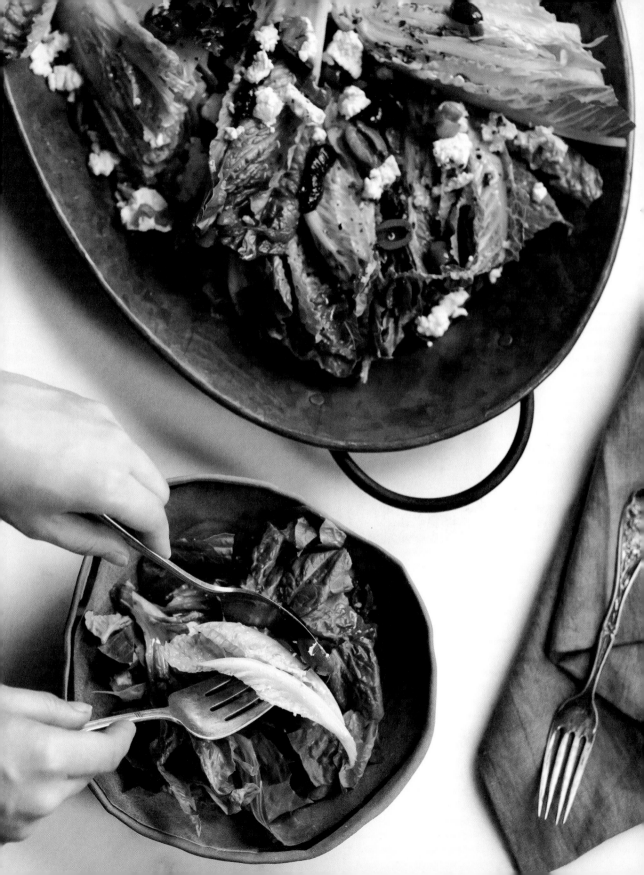

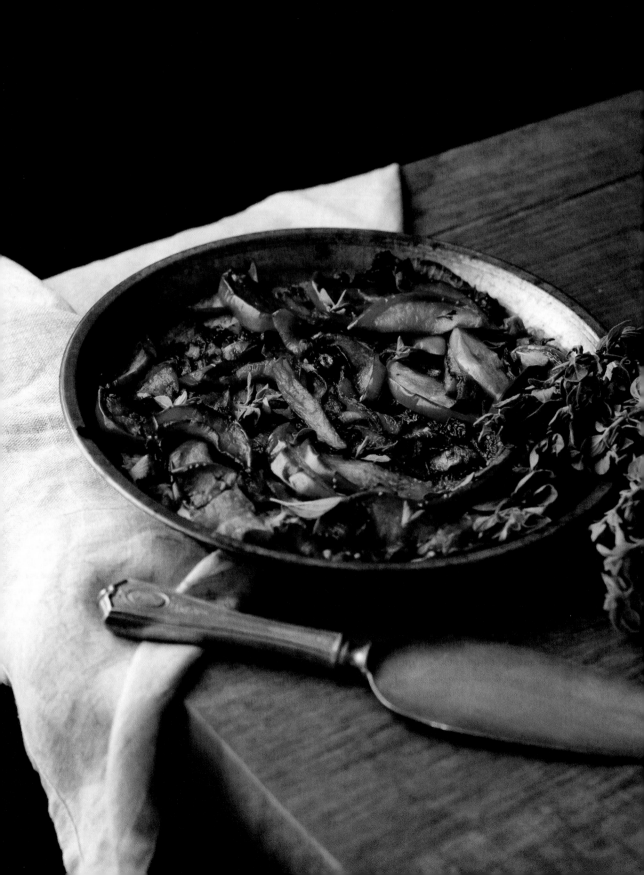

This savory tart with a fat-rich crust will make pie and tart lovers swoon. But don't worry, it's not sinful since it is make from good-quality fats, such as the kinds found in nuts. This crust is also quite versatile and can be topped with a variety of superfoods, such as cooked mushrooms, artichokes, or kale.

SAVORY APPLE
Onion Tart

Line an 8-inch round baking pan with parchment paper, cutting the paper to fit snugly in the base. Place the butter in the freezer for 30 minutes while you prep the filling. Heat the olive oil in a large skillet, preferably cast iron, over medium heat. Add the apples, onion, oregano, and garlic salt and cook, stirring occasionally, for 10 to 15 minutes, or until the apples and onion are well browned.

Meanwhile, preheat the oven to 375°F.

In a food processor, combine the frozen butter, flour, walnuts, and salt. Process until the walnuts are finely ground into the flour, about 15 seconds. Add the ice water and pulse briefly, just until the water is distributed evenly and the dough begins to come together into large pieces. Turn out the dough into the prepared baking dish. Use a spatula to press the dough evenly into the bottom of the pan. Bake for 15 to 20 minutes, or until the edges of the crust turn golden brown. Top with the cooked apples and onions. Sprinkle with the goat cheese and bake for 5 to 10 minutes, or until the cheese is melted. Cut into six wedges and serve warm or at room temperature.

SERVES 8

8 tablespoons (1 stick/4 ounces) unsalted grass-fed butter, or frozen vegan butter spread, cubed

2 tablespoons olive oil

2 apples, cored and thinly sliced

1 sweet onion, thinly sliced

1 teaspoon dried oregano

1 teaspoon garlic salt

1 cup gluten-free multipurpose flour

¾ cup walnut pieces

¼ teaspoon salt

3 tablespoons ice water

4 ounces goat cheese or cashew cheese, crumbled

---

per serving
331 *calories*
25 g (11 g) *fat (sat)*
23 g *carbs*
6 g *sugar*
2 g *fiber*
6 g *protein*
317 mg *sodium*

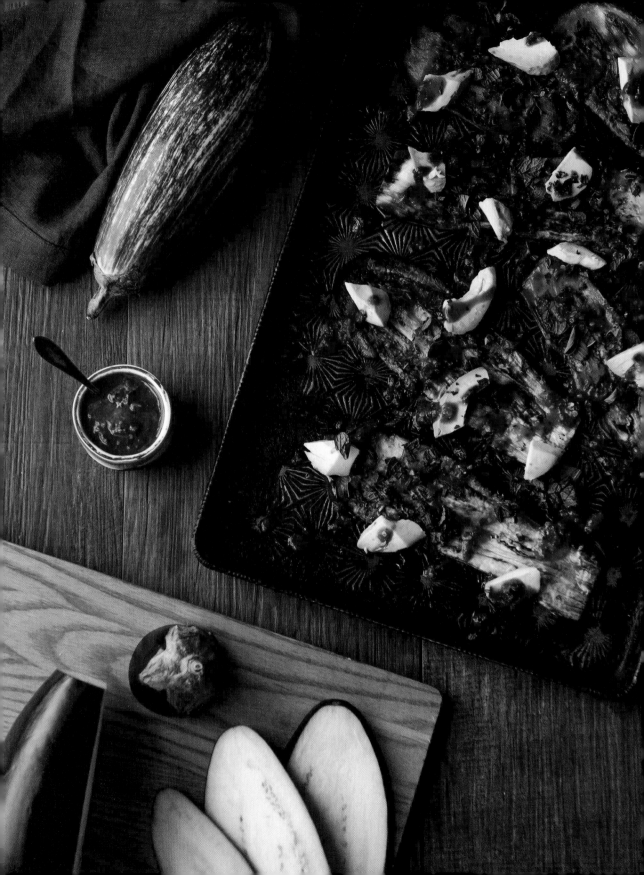

Pass on the oily fried eggplant and learn this special technique to cook soft, sensual, fiber-rich eggplant minus the grease. Salting the eggplant first helps draw out some of the bitter juices while softening it a bit before cooking. Harissa, a north African chili paste, makes a crave-worthy sauce when mixed with fresh herbs and lime juice. To make it a meal, pair the eggplant with your choice of grain or cauliflower rice.

HARISSA-
Spiced Eggplant

SERVES 4

Using a serrated bread knife, trim and discard the tops of the eggplants. Cut the eggplants lengthwise into ¼-inch-thick slices. Spread out on paper towels or tea towels on the countertop and sprinkle with ½ teaspoon of the salt. Let rest for 30 minutes to allow the bitter juices to form on the tops of the slices. Wipe off the juices with paper towels.

Coat two large skillets with cooking spray and heat over medium heat. Add the eggplant slices and cook, covered, for 5 to 7 minutes, or until the eggplant starts to brown. Coat the tops with a thin layer of cooking spray and flip, cooking for 5 minutes more, or until the eggplant starts to soften. Lower the heat to low while you prepare the sauce.

In a jar that holds more than a pint, combine the oil, tomato paste, harissa, lime juice, red chili flakes, mint, oregano, black pepper, and remaining ½ teaspoon of salt. Add 2 cups of water, close the jar, and shake to combine. Alternatively, place the same ingredients in a bowl and whisk to combine. Drizzle the sauce over the eggplant and garnish with the remaining mint and oregano. Top with avocado and serve immediately.

2 pounds purple or white eggplant, such as Italian or Japanese

1 teaspoon salt

Olive oil cooking spray

2 tablespoon sesame, coconut, or olive oil

2 tablespoons tomato paste

1 teaspoon harissa paste

Juice of ½ lime (1 tablespoon)

1 to 3 teaspoons crushed red chile flakes

¼ cup chopped fresh mint, plus 4 sprigs for garnish

1 tablespoon finely chopped fresh oregano, plus 2 sprigs for garnish

¼ teaspoon freshly ground black pepper

2 ripe Hass avocados, pitted, peeled, and sliced or diced

◇

per serving
209 *calories*
16 g (2 g) *fat (sat)*
19 g *carbs*
6 g *sugar*
11 g *fiber*
4 g *protein*
652 mg *sodium*

◇

Want a healthy and delicious appetizer for your guests to munch on while you finish up cooking the main dish? This easy platter has you covered. It is a boon for gut health since it contains a whopping 9 grams of fiber (a third of your RDA needs). And it's also a perfect dish to serve when entertaining family and friends—nourishing your soul as well as your body!

Hummus Platter
WITH APPLES AND HERB OIL

SERVES 6

GARLIC HUMMUS

2 garlic cloves

½ teaspoon salt

1 (14.5-ounce) can chickpeas, well drained

⅓ cup tahini

¼ to ⅓ cup warm water

Juice of 1 lemon

HERB OIL

½ cup fresh mint

½ cup fresh basil

¼ cup olive oil

1 teaspoon mild or hot paprika

1 (14.5-ounce) can black olives, drained

2 tart apples, such as Granny Smith, cored and thinly sliced

2 red bell peppers, seeded and cut into wedges

1 cucumber, thinly sliced

Prepare the garlic hummus: Place the garlic and salt in a food processor and finely chop. Add the chickpeas, tahini, ¼ cup of the water, and lemon juice and process until smooth. Add the additional water if the hummus isn't very smooth. Transfer the hummus to a serving platter.

Prepare the herb oil: Rinse out the food processor, then place the mint and basil in the bowl of the processor and process until finely chopped. Add the olive oil and paprika and process again until smooth. Drizzle the herb oil over the hummus.

To serve, arrange the olives, apples, peppers, and cucumber on the platter around the hummus.

per serving
366	calories
21 g (3 g)	fat (sat)
38 g	carbs
13 g	sugar
10 g	fiber
10 g	protein
521 mg	sodium

THE SUPERFOOD ALCHEMY COOKBOOK

Latkes aren't just for Hanukkah. They can also be a fun way to get more veggies into your diet at any time of year. This version features apples and sweet potatoes, which lend an irresistible sweetness to the dish. For a healthier alternative to the usual sour cream, serve these with plain Greek or coconut yogurt; they're also excellent with Cardamom-Spiced Applesauce (page 100).

SPICED APPLE AND
Sweet Potato Latkes

SERVES 4

Place the sweet potato, apple, scallions, eggs, Parmesan, pepper, cinnamon, cardamom, and ¼ teaspoon of the salt in a large bowl. Stir well to combine. Sprinkle the flour over the top of the mixture and toss well.

Heat 1 tablespoon of the oil in a large skillet, preferably cast iron, over medium-low heat. Using two forks, gather about ¼ cup of the latke mixture, drop it onto the skillet, and mash it down to flatten. Repeat until the skillet is full, spacing the mounds about 1 inch apart. Cook for 4 to 5 minutes, or until crisp, then flip and cook for 2 to 3 minutes more.

Repeat with the remaining batter and oil until all the latkes are cooked. Sprinkle with the remaining ¼ teaspoon of salt and serve immediately with yogurt for garnish.

1 sweet potato, peeled and grated

1 apple, cored and grated

2 scallions or ½ sweet onion, chopped

2 large eggs

2 tablespoons grated Parmesan cheese, or 1 tablespoon nutritional yeast

¼ teaspoon freshly ground black pepper

¼ teaspoon ground cinnamon

¼ teaspoon ground cardamom

½ teaspoon salt

1 tablespoon gluten-free multipurpose flour, or 1½ teaspoons cornstarch

2 tablespoons olive oil

½ cup plain Greek or coconut yogurt

3	*latkes*
363	*calories*
20 g (4 g)	*fat (sat)*
32 g	*carbs*
15 g	*sugar*
5 g	*fiber*
16 g	*protein*
795 mg	*sodium*

95

HEIRLOOM TOMATO AND
Tulsi Soup

SERVES 4

3 tablespoons olive oil

3 garlic cloves

1 pound heirloom tomatoes, quartered

½ teaspoon salt

¼ teaspoon freshly ground black pepper

1 quart brewed tulsi tea

2 tablespoons fresh rosemary, chopped

2 tablespoons fresh oregano, chopped

1 teaspoon mild paprika

1 avocado, pitted, peeled, and sliced (optional)

Heat 2 tablespoons of the oil in a large stockpot over medium heat. Add the garlic and cook until the garlic is golden, 1 to 2 minutes. Carefully add the tomatoes, salt, and pepper. Cook for 4 to 5 minutes, allowing the tomatoes to release their liquid. Add the tea and cook for 10 minutes more, or until the tomatoes start to break apart. Blend the soup right in the pot, using an immersion blender, or in batches in a blender.

Drizzle with the remaining tablespoon of oil. Sprinkle with the rosemary, oregano, and paprika and serve immediately, topped with the avocado (if using).

NOTE: To brew the tea, pour 1 quart of boiling water over three or four tulsi tea bags or 4 teaspoons of dried tulsi in an infuser. Allow to steep for at least 5 minutes, then remove the tulsi. It's not necessary to let the tea cool before adding it to this recipe.

	per serving
176	calories
16 g (2 g)	fat (sat)
9 g	carbs
7 g	sugar
4 g	fiber
2 g	protein
300 mg	sodium

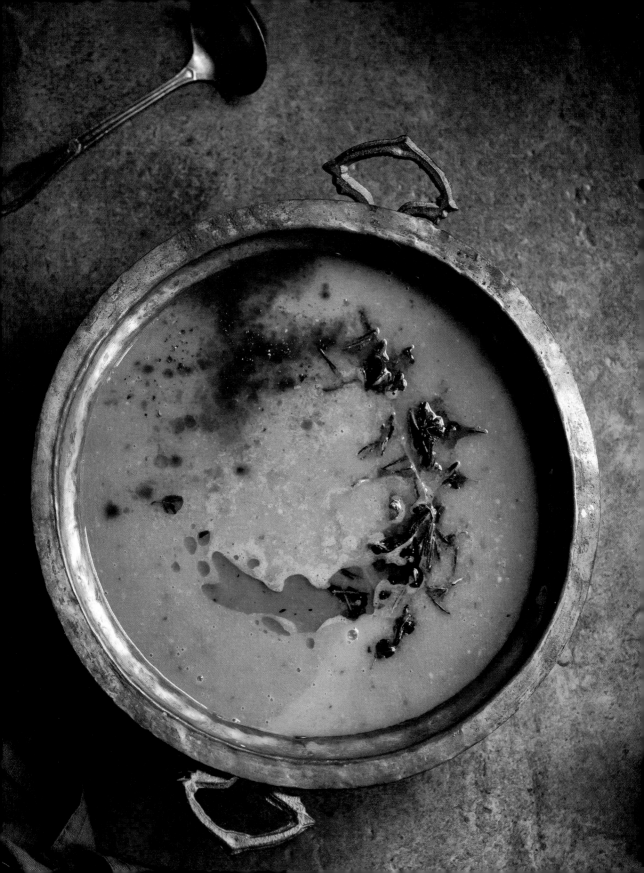

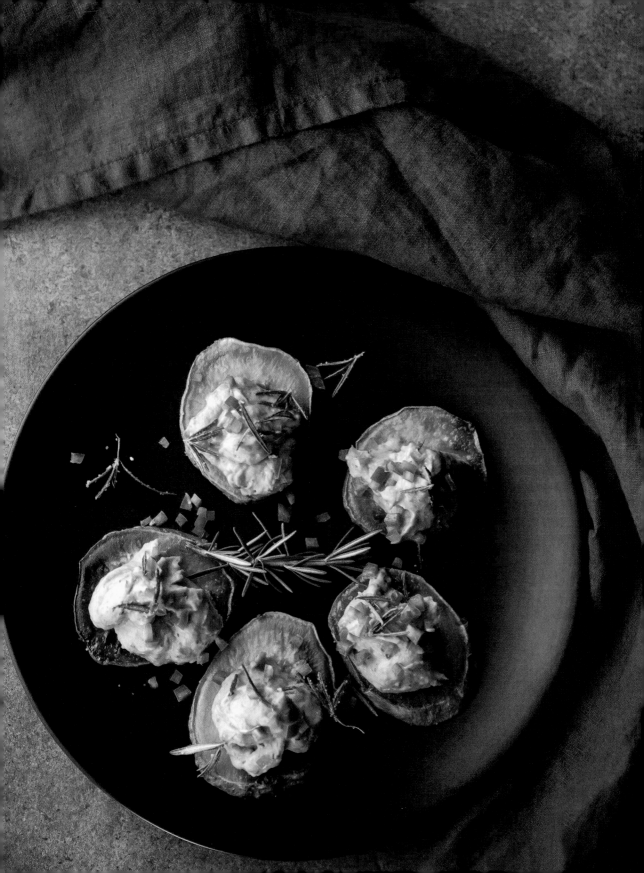

Guacamole is a beloved dip and a perfect accompaniment for nearly any Mexican dish. This nontraditional version incorporates apples for a refreshing tartness, and to boost the health of your microbiome, since apples contain pectin, a prebiotic food that feeds gut good bugs your defense against obesity and other inflammatory disorders.

Apple Guacamole
WITH SWEET POTATO CRISPS

Preheat the oven to 400°F. Using a serrated knife, cut the potatoes into ⅛-inch-thick pieces lengthwise. Heat two large, ovenproof skillets over medium heat. Heat a tablespoon of the oil in each skillet, then add the potatoes. Cook for 4 to 5 minutes, or until the potatoes start to crisp. Turn them and cook for 4 to 5 minutes more. Slide the skillets into the oven and roast for 10 to 15 minutes, or until the potatoes are cooked through. While the potatoes are roasting, prepare the guacamole.

Place the apple, cilantro, jalapeño, and salt in a food processor. Process to finely chop. Cut the avocados in half, pit, and scoop out the flesh. Add the avocado and lime juice to the food processor and pulse ten to fifteen times, or until creamy. Serve with the potato crisps.

SERVES 4

1 pound sweet potatoes (about 2 potatoes)

2 tablespoons olive oil

1 Granny Smith apple, peeled, cored, and quartered

½ cup fresh cilantro leaves and stems

1 jalapeño pepper, stemmed and quartered

1 teaspoon salt

4 ripe Hass avocados

Juice of 1 lime

---

per serving
391 *calories*
28 g (4 g) *fat (sat)*
38 g *carbs*
7 g *sugar*
14 g *fiber*
5 g *protein*
612 mg *sodium*

Applesauce is a homey, fiber-rich side dish or dessert that you can make in large batches and take on the go. To make this dish extra-special, add a drop of food-grade essential oil, such orange, cardamom, or cinnamon.

CARDAMOM-SPICED
Applesauce

MAKES 3 CUPS APPLESAUCE

4 large Macintosh apples, peeled, cored, and chopped into 1-inch chunks

½ teaspoon ground cardamom

¼ teaspoon ground cinnamon

¼ teaspoon freshly ground nutmeg

1 teaspoon stevia (optional)

Place the apples in a medium-size saucepan with enough water to cover. Place over medium heat and simmer for 10 to 12 minutes, or until the apples are tender and starting to break apart. Add the spices and stevia (if using), stir well, and serve warm, or chill in an airtight container for at least 1 hour before serving.

¾ cup
183 calories
0 g (0 g) fat (sat)
26 g carbs
19 g sugar
5 g fiber
1 g protein
2 mg sodium

Pineapple contains bromelain, an enzyme that works as a natural digestive aid, since it breaks down proteins and debris that can be lingering in the lining of the intestines. Aloe vera juice soothes those membranes throughout the body and pairs well with tropical pineapple as they hail from a similar climate. When shopping for aloe vera juice, look for unsweetened options with no added flavorings.

PINEAPPLE
Cucumber Slushie

Place the pineapple, aloe juice, cucumber, mint, and ice cubes in a blender and blend until smooth. Serve immediately.

SERVES 2

2 cups cubed pineapple

1 cup aloe juice

½ large cucumber

2 tablespoons fresh mint leaves

4 ice cubes

2 cups	
159	calories
0 g (0 g)	fat (sat)
40 g	carbs
33 g	sugar
3 g	fiber
2 g	protein
5 mg	sodium

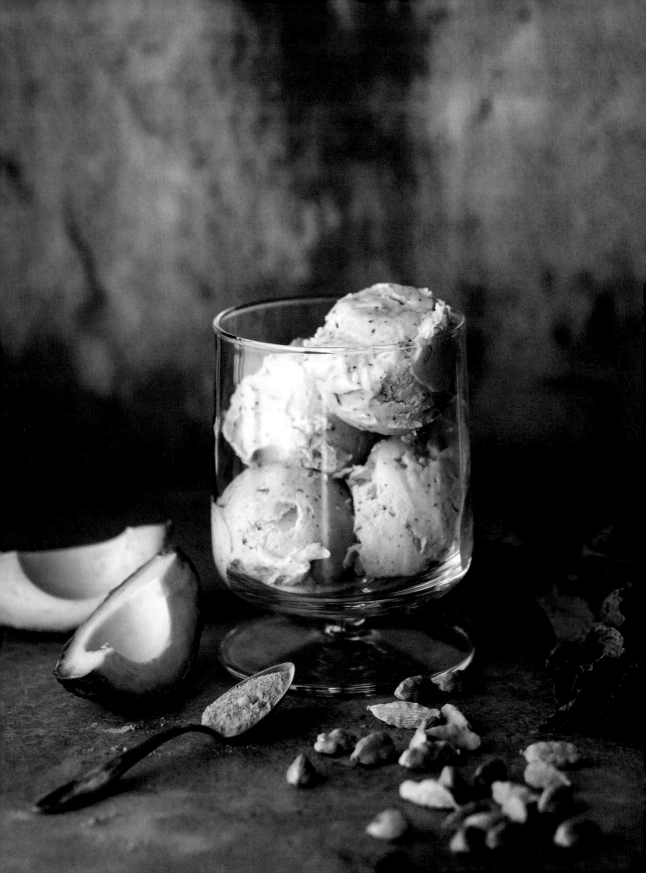

Matcha tea is a superfood that can boost metabolism and is packed with antioxidants. Green tea lovers will adore this sweet, rich treat that gets its ice cream–like flavor from avocado's antioxidant-rich fats. Avocados may seem like a sinful fruit, but they provide plenty of nourishment for your gut and make an excellent swap for heavy cream in dessert preparation. Avocados are rarely ripe when you buy them, so plan to store them on the windowsill or a basket two to three days, or until they are soft to the touch.

MINTY AVOCADO
Green Tea Ice Cream

MAKES 2½ CUPS ICE CREAM; SERVES 5

Place the avocado, mint, matcha, cardamom, coconut milk, honey or agave or stevia, vanilla, xanthan gum (if using), and salt in a blender and process until smooth. Transfer to an ice-cream machine and process according to the manufacturer's instructions.

If you don't have an ice-cream maker, place the mixture in an airtight container and freeze for 1 hour. Remove from the freezer and scrape the mixture with a fork to fluff. Return the mixture to the freezer and freeze for at least 1 more hour before serving.

1 large, ripe Haas avocado, pitted and peeled

½ cup fresh mint

2 teaspoons powdered matcha tea

½ teaspoon ground cardamom

1 (14.5 ounce) can coconut milk

⅓ cup honey or agave nectar, or 3 tablespoons stevia

2 teaspoons pure vanilla extract

½ teaspoon xanthan gum (optional)

Pinch of salt

½ cup	
177	calories
8 g (3 g)	fat (sat)
26 g	carbs
22 g	sugar
4 g	fiber
2 g	protein
139 mg	sodium

Essential Oil Preparations and Rituals for Separation

DIFFUSER OIL BLEND FOR CENTERING

Looking for a fast way to feel more confident? Deep breathing can stimulate the vagus nerve, the longest nerve in the body, which stretches from the brain down into the gut. The vagus nerve controls the motor functions of your stomach and how well food passes from your stomach by contracting the muscles in a smooth flow and ensuring that food isn't lingering too long the stomach. But what happens in "vagus," doesn't always stay in vagus, meaning that if this nerve is uptight, your digestion will be off kilter. Stimulating the vagus nerve is also known to release a substance that slows your heart rate. So, centering yourself, by enjoying a few moments of this calming aromatherapy oil blend while taking deep breaths, is a fast way to release nervous or fearful energy.

3 drops cardamom essential oil

3 drops lime essential oil

1 drop lemongrass oil

Fill your essential oil diffuser with water according to the diffuser instructions. Add the oils and turn on the mister.

DIFFUSER OIL BLEND FOR SELF-CONFIDENCE

If you're feeling unnerved, you can get more than butterflies in your stomach; your digestion can take a huge hit since your parasympathetic nervous system puts a hold on all gut functions. This balancing blend of oils will help you to release feelings of nervousness and give you an overall confidence boost.

2 drops cinnamon essential oil

2 drops oregano essential oil

Fill your essential oil diffuser with water according to the diffuser instructions. Add the oils and turn on the mister.

HAPPY HOLIDAY DIFFUSER BLEND

Part of feeling confident is embracing the joy of socializing. This oil blend is perfect for fall and winter holidays since it smells like baking cookies.

2 drops cardamom essential oil

2 drops lemon or orange essential oil

1 drop nutmeg essential oil

Fill your essential oil diffuser with water according to the diffuser instructions. Add the oils and turn on the mister.

CLARY SAGE MAKEUP REMOVER

Having clear skin can instantly boost confidence and make you feel radiant! Removing makeup at the end of the night is key because oils in makeup can block pores and create acne. Proper cleansing at the end of the night also can help remove environmental pollution from your skin that gathers during the day.

2 tablespoons aloe vera gel

2 tablespoons witch hazel

1 teaspoon liquid castile soap

1 teaspoon jojoba or sweet almond oil

1 drop clary sage oil (optional)

Place the aloe vera gel, witch hazel, castile soap, jojoba oil, and clary sage oil (if using) in a small bowl along with 1 tablespoon of cold water and stir well to combine.

VANILLA CARDAMOM ROLLERBALL COLOGNE

This simply delicious scent will remind you of the smell of freshly baked donuts with a hint of spice. Since it's made with oil, it can double as a scented moisturizer for hands or elbows.

MAKES 1 1/2 OUNCES

2 tablespoons jojobo or sweet almond oil

10 drops cardamom essential oil

5 drops orange essential oil

2 drops sandalwood oil

½ teaspoon pure vanilla extract or 2 drops vanilla essential oil

Place the oil, cardamom, and vanilla extract or essential oil in a measuring cup with a spout. Mix well with a spatula and transfer to a rollerball bottle. Faster the rollerball top and apply to neck and pulse points.

CARDAMOM HONEY BODY WASH

Bathing and showering are relaxing, necessary rituals, but do you know your standard cake of soap can greatly affect the health of the good bacteria that inhabit your body, inside your gut and out? Skip the antibacterial soap and wipes that contain triclosan, which also wipes out your good flora, and use this homemade natural soap made with a castile base instead.

MAKES 1 CUP BODY WASH

⅔ cup liquid castile soap

⅓ cup honey

5 drops cardamom essential oil

5 drops chamomile or lavender essential oil

1 teaspoon pure vanilla extract

¼ teaspoon ground cinnamon

Place the castile soap, honey, essential oils, vanilla, and cinnamon in a small bowl. Gently whisk to combine. Transfer to a squirt bottle or glass mason jar. Use 2 to 3 tablespoons per shower or bath.

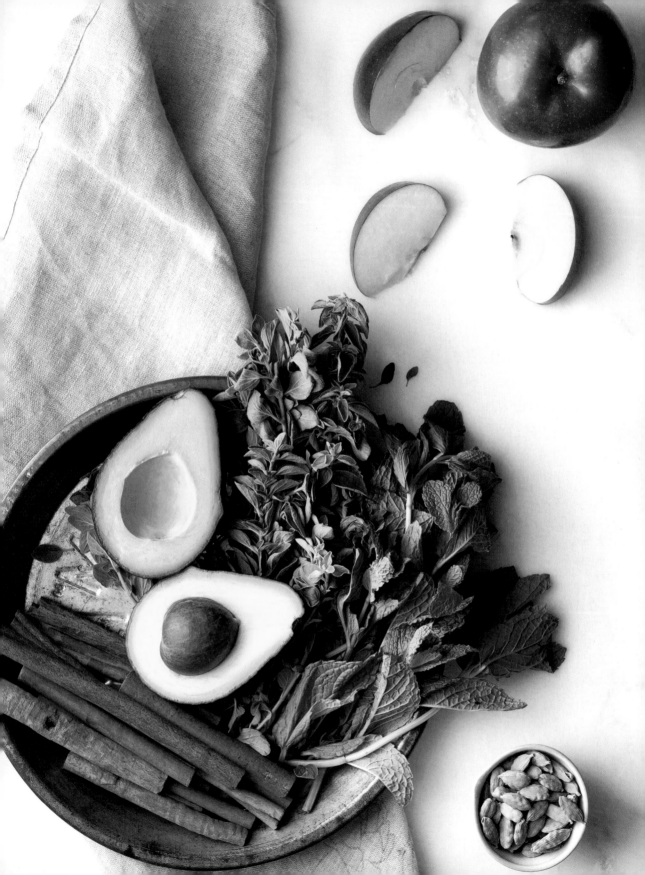

DETOX GREEN TEA CARDAMOM MASK

Double up on this medicinal plant that softens skin when you make this mask while sipping a cup of green tea. Green tea contains polyphenols that curb harmful bacteria while allowing good flora to flourish, which is helpful for gut health. If you don't savory the scent of cardamom oil, feel free to omit it or select an essential oil that is safe for your face, such as lavender or frankincense.

MAKES 1 MASK

1 tablespoon powdered matcha green tea

1 tablespoon bentonite clay

1 teaspoon cider vinegar

2 drops cardamom essential oil

Place the matcha, bentonite clay, vinegar, and cardamom oil in a small bowl along with 2 tablespoons of water. Mix with a spatula until a thick paste starts to form. Add 2 tablespoons of warm water and stir again; the mixture will foam. Apply to your face and allow to dry, until the mask tightens on your face and is a light shade of green, 10 to 15 minutes. Remove with a washcloth and warm water. Moisturize as usual.

WARM OREGANO WATER

Candida is a fungus (a form of yeast) that normally helps up with digestion living in small amounts in your mouth and intestines. It's not a problem when in balance, but when your microbiome and good gut bugs aren't operating at 100 percent, *Candida* can take over, causing a host of problems, such as brain fog, fatigue, and regular vaginal yeast infections. Processed sugar, white processed flour, trans fats from fast food, and gluten can lead to overgrowth. If you have *Candida*, work with your doctor's guidance and pair up this easy oregano remedy.

SERVES 1

4 ounces warm, filtered water

2 drops food-grade oregano essential oil

Place the warm water in a cup or mug. Stir in the oregano oil and drink on an empty stomach, once a day.

Probiotic Basics

If you want to give your microbiome a boost, you can always opt for a probiotic supplement, a smart way to reseed your gut with helpful flora. Next follow the step of removing bad foods from your diet and replacing them with prebiotic foods featured in this chapter, such as apples. Probiotics are generally safe and are even recommended for children and pets, though you can consult your doctor before taking them if you have concerns. If you suffer from more severe GI issues, probiotics may not have a noticeable effect, since such disorders, such as IBS, leaky gut, and small intestine bacterial overgrowth (SIBO) mean that you must clean out the harmful bacteria first with an illumination diet before a reintroduction of probiotic bacteria can flourish.

Healing Stone Therapy
Tigereye, citrine, and pyrite are all healing crystals for this area. While practicing any of the meditations featured in this book, you can rest one of these crystals in your belly button. Carry one of these crystals with you when you need a confidence boost, on days when giving a public speech, or when interviewing for a new job.

Earth Meditation

Part of feeling more confident is trusting your body to heal itself, separate out what isn't needed, and realizing that many of the things you need to heal already flourish in your environment, such as healing plants and even microbes that live in the soil and in our guts. This meditation crosses the science of the microbiome with spiritual visualization, to give you a deeper understanding of the forces at work when it comes to your health. This meditation can also feel quite grounding and supportive, since you'll stimulate the vagus nerve (see page 104) with deep breathing, and connect with the solid life-giving energy of the earth.

We are deeply linked both physically and spiritually to earth energy. Physically we draw all of our nourishment from the earth in the form of nutrient-rich plants and animals, and the earth's minerals, such as salt, iron, magnesium, and calcium, play a vital role in our health. On the spiritual level, we are subconsciously and energetically linked to our earth because we are born from her. A deeper relationship with the earth can help you feel more alive, more connected to your body, as well as safer and stronger—she is the mother and has so much to give to us. This meditation helps you draw on earth energy to nourish the spirit.

If the weather allows, you may want to do this meditation outdoors in the grass to feel a more immediate connection to the earth (not to mention, soil microbes are great for you—the dirt is rich in vital microorganisms that can contribute to our gut bacteria and may be good for mental health).

Find a comfortable seat. Start by breathing in steadily and slowly to move energy around your body and open up your lungs. Take slow breaths in through your nose to the count of four, imagine that your stomach area is "drinking" in air as you breathe in deeply. Exhale slowly to the count of four. Inhale and imagine your stomach slowly rising as it expands. Imagine your stomach cavity forming a perfectly round balloon. Slowly exhale through your nose to a count of four. Repeat twice more, keeping the image of a rounding balloon in your mind as you breathe.

As you continue this conscious breath, begin to sense your seat and legs on the floor. Feel them firmly rooting toward the ground. Imagine actual roots extending deep into the earth, seeking nourishment.

As you breathe in, take this moment to feel grateful for that support you receive from the earth and her abundant soil, day in and day out. As you send down roots, feel them tapping into the earth's strong, rich energy. As you feel this primal energy rise from your roots into your body, send a special thank-you back down through the root. Continue to breathe in and out to the count of four, sending your thank-you to the earth as you relax and allow the energy to absorb throughout the body. When you are ready to end the meditation, take a slow breath in and out to the count of ten, and slowly open your eyes.

Separation Breathing Technic

Air is the alchemical element for separation and learning how to breath more deeply can not only make you feel more confident by improving your blood flow and oxygenating your brain better, but also reduce "shallow upper chest" breathing that can trigger stress hormones.

Find a comfortable seat on the floor or in a chair. Sit with a tall spine. Rest your left palm on your left knee, moving your right hand toward the nose. Use the right thumb, softly close the right nostril, and inhale as slowly as you can through the left nostril, expanding the belly, then the rib cage, and finally the upper chest. Then close it with your ring finger (both nostrils are closed). Pause for 30 seconds. Open and exhale slowly through the right nostril only, keeping the exhale as slow and quiet as possible.

With the right nostril still open, inhale slowly, expanding the belly, then rib cage, and finally upper chest then close it with the thumb. Pause for 30 seconds. Exhale through the left nostril. Once your exhalation is complete, inhale through the left. Pause before moving to the right.

Repeat this pattern ten times for beginners, twenty times for a more advanced breathing practice. Release the right hand to the right knee and breathe normally. Set a goal to do this practice daily, to reduce stress and better oxygenate the body.

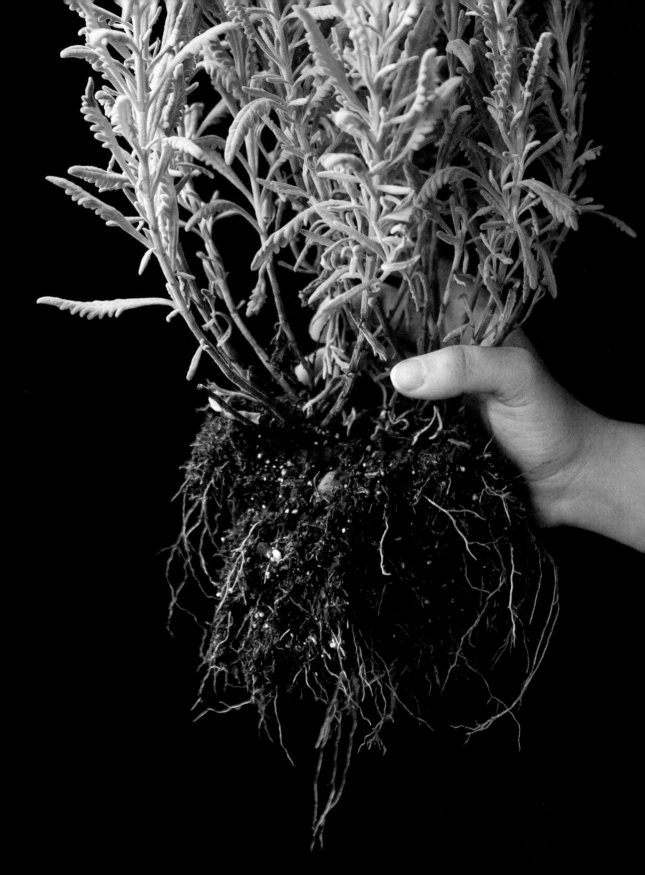

Conjunction

BALANCING ENERGIES AND HEALING THE HEART

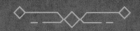

Conjunction is a great operation to work with, since it focuses on the heart center and on learning to love the real you.

Are you ready for love or just want to learn to love yourself more? Conjunction is a great operation to work with, since it focuses on the heart center and on learning to love the real you. Conjunction in alchemy is the idea of "two celestial bodies coming together"—sounds pretty exciting, right? In old alchemy texts, this operation is often portrayed as romantic, with imagery of a handsome couple, such as a king and queen, united or embracing. But for us, conjunction is less about the idea of romantic love and more about love in a broader spiritual sense. It is concerned with unifying right and left brain, bringing together creativity and logic, finding a balance of the feminine and masculine energies inside, and loving yourself and others.

The recipes and therapies in this chapter correspond to the energy center surrounding the heart.

Your heart can take a hit not only with emotional pain but also from diet and stress; in addition to nutrients for the heart, superfoods for this chapter also help with processing fats (fat in the blood and excess fat on the body puts your heart at serious risk). Detoxing your diet by incorporating plant-based foods is such an easy way to care for your heart, your circulatory system, and your body in general. In addition to the recipes here, to rev up your heart health, add some form of cardio exercise to your routine. The options are nearly endless: kickboxing, dancing, spinning, and hot yoga are all options if you're not enamored of running.

Superfoods, Herbs, and Essential Oils for the Heart

CRUCIFEROUS VEGETABLES (INCLUDING BROCCOLI, CAULIFLOWER, AND KALE): Cruciferous vegetables have special fibers that latch onto fats during the digestion process and whisk them away before they can build up in your blood. Cruciferous vegetables are all high in vitamin C, widely researched for its ability to protect the lining of blood vessels.

ALMONDS: Delightfully crunchy, these satisfying superfood nuts contain a winning combo of heart-protective nutrients, including vitamin E, fiber, and monounsaturated fats, which may work together to lower LDL, the "bad" cholesterol. Almonds' slightly bitter skins have the highest antioxidant load, so be sure to shop for whole almonds with the skins on.

RASPBERRIES: Tart, slightly sweet raspberries are ubiquitous in Valentine's Day treats and also happen to be a superfood for your physical heart. They have very high levels of three must-have nutrients for heart health—fiber, vitamin C, and manganese—delivering over 30 percent of your RDA of all three in just 1 cup.

GREEN TEA: This brew with medicinal benefits can be added right into recipes, or enjoyed as a beverage with or after meals. Catechins, a group of polyphenols, the healing compounds in green tea, have been shown to increase both fat oxidation and energy expenditure.

BASIL AND BASIL OIL: Basil is high in vitamin K, needed for proper blood clotting. Basil oil contains the same properties of the food in condensed form and is delicious used in foods, 1 to 2 drops per recipe in place of dried herbs. Basil is high in antibacterial compounds, such as eugenol and limonene, which can help combat pathogens that may cause heart disease, such as *E-coli*.

HAWTHORN BERRIES: Used by herbalists for heart ailments, specifically high blood pressure and heart arrhythmia, bitter hawthorn berries come from a shrub in the rose family. They are incredibly high in antioxidants, along with many other compounds that help protect blood vessels, zap free radicals, and slow down general wear and tear on the heart.

ROSE ESSENTIAL OIL: Sweet and fragrant, rose is recognized worldwide as a healing plant for the heart on an emotional level. Since rose essential oil can be very strong and floral, you'll find it blended with other oils to balance it.

GERANIUM ESSENTIAL OIL: Geranium has a light vegetal scent mixed with a hint of floral, making it a fresh light lift to your diffuser blends.

ANGELICA ESSENTIAL OIL: A plant in the same family as celery and carrot, angelica has lacy white blooms reminiscent of Queen Anne's lace. Traditionally used as a nervine, it's included in this chapter as an aromatherapy option to soothe heartbreak.

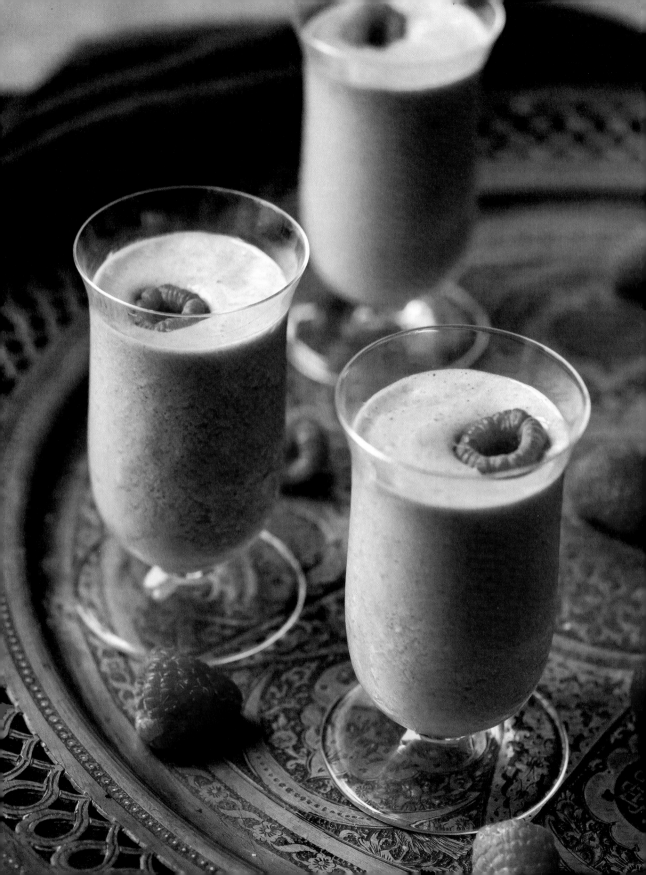

Sensual ruby red is the color that comes to mind when we think of both love and heart health, and the plant world agrees! Red pigments in plants, mainly anthocyanins, are found in such superfoods as hawthorn berries and raspberries, and they do wonders for the heart.

HAWTHORN BERRY TEA
Raspberry Smoothie

SERVES 2

Place the raspberries, protein powder, tea, honey, cinnamon, and ice cubes in a blender and process until smooth. Divide between two cups and serve immediately.

NOTE: To brew the tea, pour 1 cup of boiling water over one hawthorn berry tea bag or 1 to 2 teaspoons of dried hawthorn berries in an infuser. Steep for 5 to 10 minutes, then remove the berries or tea bag. Let the tea cool completely before using it in this recipe.

2 cups fresh or frozen raspberries

⅔ cup protein powder or Greek yogurt

1 cup strongly brewed hawthorn berry tea

1 tablespoon honey, or 1 teaspoon stevia

½ teaspoon ground cinnamon

8 ice cubes

per serving
197 *calories*
3 g (1 g) *fat (sat)*
30 g *carbs*
16 g *sugar*
11 g *fiber*
20 g *protein*
82 mg *sodium*

115

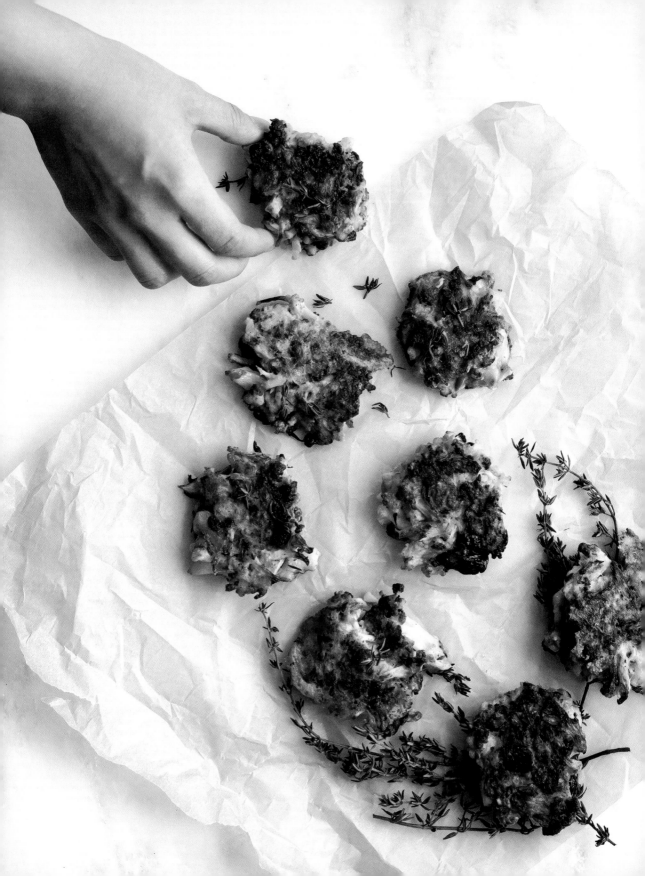

These fritters are an incredibly satisfying finger food, made from heart-nourishing superfoods cauliflower and almond, held together by egg, a superfood for the whole body, rich in all eight essential amino acids. If you don't do eggs, you can skip them and cook this up as a cauliflower hash instead. Serve warm, right out of the skillet, or make a double batch up to a few hours ahead for a brunch buffet.

CAULIFLOWER
Almond Fritters

SERVES 4

Place 2 tablespoons of the olive oil in a cast-iron skillet over medium-high heat. Add the cauliflower, salt, and pepper. Cover and cook, tossing occasionally, for 8 to 10 minutes, or until the cauliflower is well browned and tender. Transfer the cauliflower to a large bowl and let cool for 5 minutes. Add the eggs, ground flaxseeds, almond flour, olives, and thyme to the cauliflower. Toss to combine, and gently mash with the spatula or fork until a chunky mixture forms. Form the mixture into patties 4 inches in diameter.

Wipe clean the cast-iron skillet used for the cauliflower. Place the remaining 2 tablespoons of olive oil in the skillet over medium-high heat. Add the patties, spaced 1 inch apart. Cook, turning once or twice, for 2 to 3 minutes, or until the fritters are cooked through.

4 tablespoons olive oil

1 head cauliflower, chopped

½ teaspoons salt

¼ teaspoon freshly ground black pepper

2 large eggs

¼ cup ground flaxseeds

½ cup almond flour

¼ cup chopped olives, such as Kalamata

2 tablespoons chopped fresh thyme leaves

per serving
306	*calories*
24 g (3 g)	*fat (sat)*
24 g	*carbs*
3 g	*sugar*
6 g	*fiber*
10 g	*protein*
419 mg	*sodium*

This glossy, emerald green salad offers a new way to enjoy the multifold health benefits of spinach. The green is full of nutrients for your heart, such as folate, a B vitamin that helps keep homocysteine, a marker for heart disease, in check. Scientists who are studying spinach in connection with heart cell regeneration note that leaf veins even resemble blood vessels in the heart.

Charred Lemon Spinach Salad
WITH THYME DRESSING

SERVES 4

Cooking spray

2 lemons, thinly sliced into rounds and seeded

¼ cup olive oil

1 shallot, minced

1 tablespoon fresh thyme leaves

1 tablespoon freshly squeezed lemon juice

1 teaspoon Dijon mustard

½ teaspoon salt

¼ teaspoon freshly ground black pepper

1 pound greens

1 avocado, pitted, peeled, and thinly sliced

Coat a cast-iron skillet with cooking spray and heat it over medium-high heat. Place lemon slices in the hot skillet in a single layer (you may have to complete this step in batches). Cook the lemon slices on one side until browned, 1 to 2 minutes. Flip and repeat so that both sides are browned, with some charred spots. Transfer the lemons to a plate and set aside. Place the olive oil, shallot, thyme, lemon juice, mustard, salt, and pepper in a large bowl and whisk well to combine. Add the greens and toss well. Top with the charred lemons and avocado and serve.

per serving
207 *calories*
19 g (3 g) *fat (sat)*
8 g *carbs*
1 g *sugar*
5 g *fiber*
4 g *protein*
413 mg *sodium*

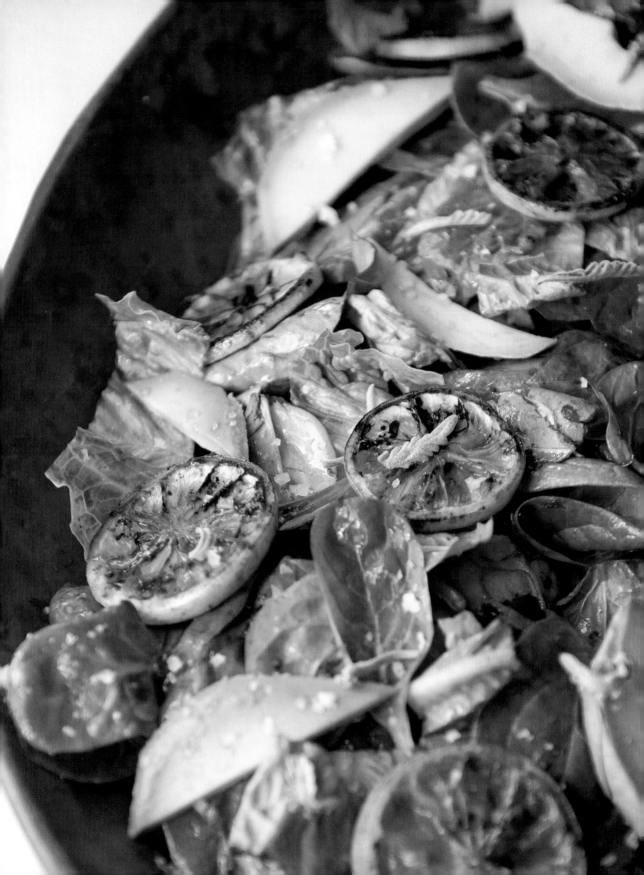

Enjoy this hearty salad in fall or winter when kale is at its sweetest after the first frost. The key to making tempting Superfood Alchemy salads is a zesty homemade dressing drizzled over a salad with different textures and even different temperatures. This recipe is a delight for the taste buds and the soul, pairing cool greens with warm roasted tomatoes spiked with cloves.

Baby Kale Salad
WITH BLACK OLIVES AND
SPICED ROASTED TOMATOES

SERVES 4

1 pound tomatoes, any variety, quartered

½ teaspoon ground cloves

¼ teaspoon salt

¼ teaspoon freshly ground black pepper

¼ cup olive oil

1 tablespoon yellow or white miso paste

1 tablespoon cider vinegar

2 teaspoons honey or agave nectar, or 1 teaspoon stevia (optional)

2 teaspoons Bragg Liquid Aminos or low-sodium tamari

1 pound baby kale

½ cup pitted black olives

¼ cup fresh basil leaves

Preheat the oven to 400ºF. Place a piece of parchment paper on a rimmed baking sheet. Spread out the tomatoes on the prepared baking sheet and sprinkle with the cloves, salt, and pepper. Drizzle with 1 tablespoon of the olive oil and toss to coat. Roast for 30 to 35 minutes, or until the tomatoes are tender. Remove from the oven and set aside to cool slightly.

Place the remaining tablespoon of oil in a large bowl along with the miso, vinegar, honey or stevia (if using), and liquid aminos and whisk well to combine. Add the kale, olives, basil leaves, and tomatoes, tossing well to combine. Serve immediately.

per serving
229 *calories*
16 g (2 g) *fat (sat)*
20 g *carbs*
8 g *sugar*
4 g *fiber*
4 g *protein*
569 mg *sodium*

Buffalo chicken was a 1960s invention that quickly established itself as a favorite in crowded sports bars across the country. This twist on the beloved bar food contains three superfood surprises: cauliflower, hot chiles in the hot sauce, and turmeric. A healthy tangy yogurt sauce replaces the usual blue cheese dressing. Serving this dish warm activates the turmeric, which is better absorbed by the body when it is served in warm foods containing fat.

TURMERIC
Buffalo Cauliflower

Preheat the oven to 400°F.

Prepare the dipping sauce: Whisk together the yogurt, mayonnaise, vinegar, mustard, and pepper in a small bowl. Cover and refrigerate while you prepare the cauliflower.

Mix together the olive oil, salt, and ½ cup of water in a large bowl. Add the cauliflower and toss until well coated. Spread out the cauliflower on a rimmed baking sheet and roast until just tender and beginning to brown, 20 to 25 minutes. Place the hot sauce, butter, tomato paste, lemon juice, and turmeric in a small saucepan over low heat and cook, whisking, for 2 to 3 minutes, or until thoroughly combined. When the cauliflower is almost fork-tender, drizzle with the hot sauce mixture and bake for an additional 10 minutes, or until tender. Sprinkle with the scallions and serve with the dipping sauce.

DIPPING SAUCE

¼ cup plain Greek or coconut yogurt

2 tablespoons mayonnaise

2 teaspoons cider vinegar

1 teaspoon Dijon mustard

¼ teaspoon freshly ground black pepper

2 tablespoons olive oil

¼ teaspoon salt

1 head cauliflower, cut into florets

⅓ cup hot sauce, such as Frank's

2 tablespoons unsalted grass-fed butter or vegan butter spread

1 tablespoon tomato paste

1 tablespoon freshly squeezed lemon juice

1 teaspoon ground turmeric

4 scallions, thinly sliced

---

per serving
187 *calories*
15 g (5 g) *fat (sat)*
10 g *carbs*
4 g *sugar*
3 g *fiber*
5 g *protein*
684 mg *sodium*

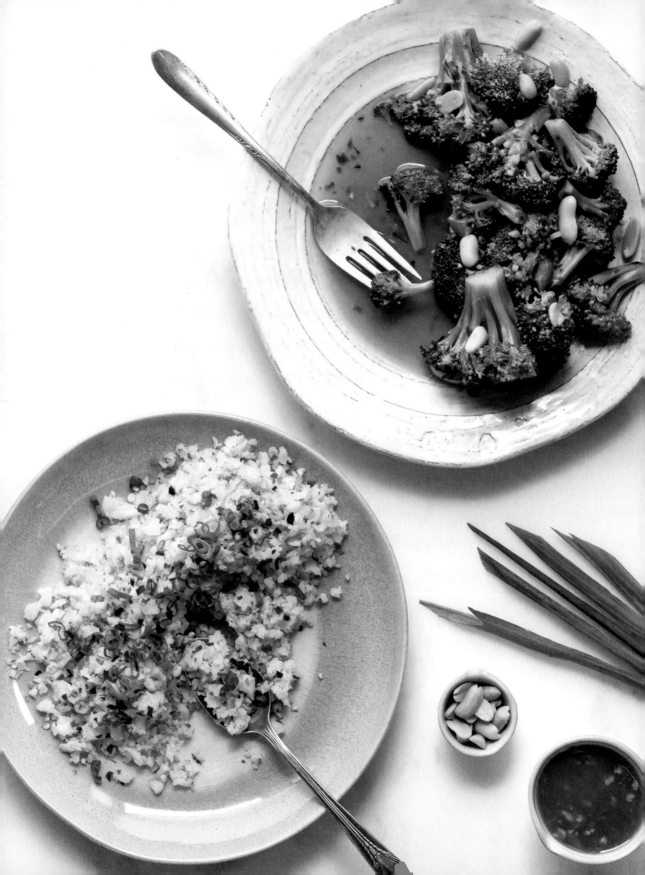

Kung Pao is a spicy peanut-studded dish that any chile pepper fan will love. Combining chiles with cauliflower is an alchemical pairing: the two foods contain cancer fighting compounds (gluconsinalate and capsaicin)—and they also happen to taste amazing together.

Kung Pao Broccoli
WITH CAULIFLOWER RICE

SERVES 4

To rice the cauliflower, place the florets in a food processor and roughly chop. You will need to do this in two or three batches. Heat 2 tablespoons of the oil in a large skillet over medium heat. Add the riced cauliflower to the skillet and cook for 2 to 3 minutes, or until tender. Set aside.

Place the stock, chiles, garlic, vinegar, tamari, ginger, honey, cornstarch, and sesame oil (if using) in a small bowl and whisk to combine. Heat the remaining 2 tablespoons of olive oil a large skillet over medium heat. Add the broccoli and cook for 6 to 8 minutes, or until the broccoli starts to soften. Reduce the heat to low and add the stock mixture. Cover and cook for 1 minute, or until the broccoli is fork-tender and a thick sauce forms. Sprinkle with the scallions and peanuts and serve immediately over the cauliflower rice.

1 head cauliflower, cut into florets

4 tablespoons olive oil

1 cup vegetable stock

8 to 10 dried red chiles, crumbled in a mortar and pestle, or 2 tablespoons red pepper flakes

2 garlic cloves, minced

1 tablespoon cider vinegar

1 tablespoon low-sodium tamari

1 tablespoon minced fresh ginger

1 tablespoon honey or agave nectar, or 1 teaspoon stevia

2 teaspoons cornstarch

1 teaspoon sesame oil (optional)

1 head broccoli, cut into florets

4 scallions, thinly sliced

¼ cup unsalted dry-roasted peanuts

per serving
262 *calories*
20 g (2 g) *fat (sat)*
17 g *carbs*
8 g *sugar*
4 g *fiber*
7 g *protein*
393 mg *sodium*

123

Love those fragrant Italian flavors of oregano, tomato, and olive oil? Then, you'll enjoy oreganata, a traditional Italian preparation that uses healing oregano as a way to flavor mild tomato-based dishes. Cooking tomatoes is a Superfood Alchemy tactic since heat increases lycopene uptake.

Stuffed Tomatoes Oreganata
WITH QUINOA

SERVES 4

1 cup uncooked quinoa or millet

1 cup pitted black olives, chopped

½ cup vegetable stock

1 tablespoon tomato paste

2 teaspoons fresh oregano, chopped

½ teaspoon salt

¼ teaspoon freshly ground black pepper

8 tomatoes (about 2 pounds)

½ cup grated Parmesan cheese, or ¼ cup nutritional yeast

2 teaspoons olive oil

Cook your grain of choice according to the package instructions. Place in a large bowl along with the olives, stock, tomato paste, oregano, salt, and pepper. Toss well.

Meanwhile, preheat the oven to 400°F. Cut off and discard the tops of the tomatoes. Scoop out the center of each tomato, discarding the watery seeds. Place the tomatoes in an 8 by 12-inch baking dish. Fill each tomato with the grain mixture and sprinkle each with a tablespoon of Parmesan and drizzle with the olive oil. Bake for 25 to 30 minutes, or until the cheese is bubbly and brown. Serve immediately.

per serving
307 *calories*
11 g (3 g) *fat (sat)*
40 g *carbs*
7 g *sugar*
7 g *fiber*
13 g *protein*
785 mg *sodium*

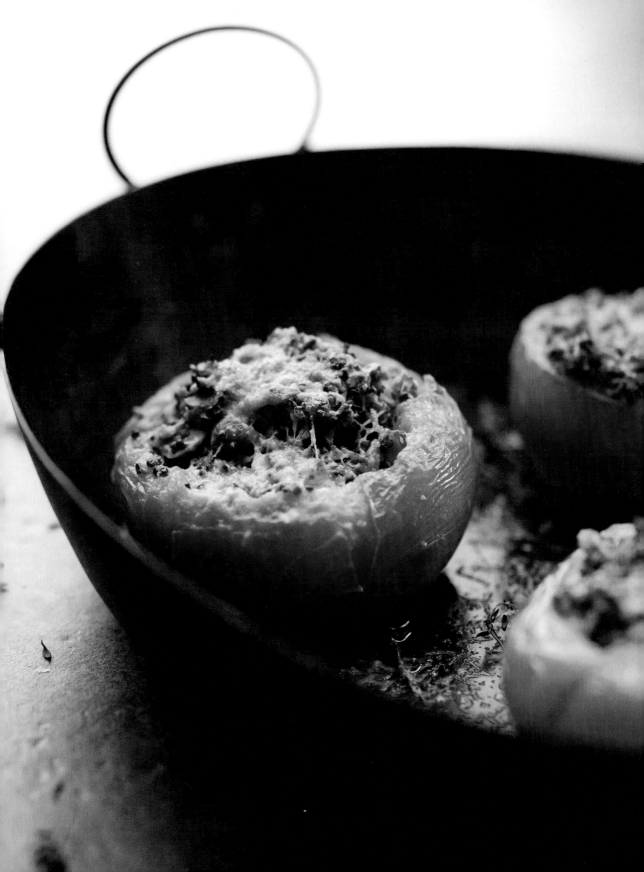

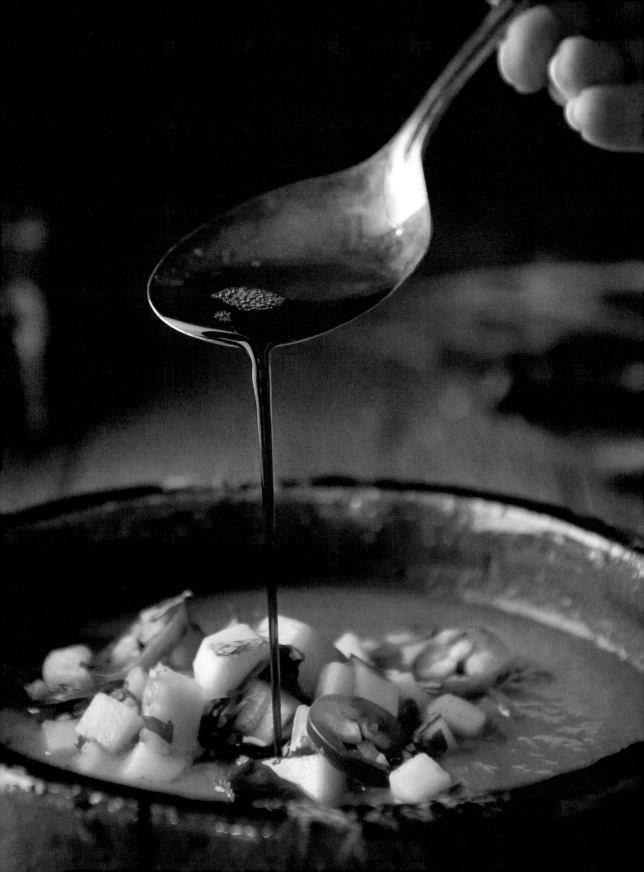

Who said pumpkin was just for making pie? This soup offers all the benefits of this fiber-rich superfood, which also contains plenty of vitamin C and potassium and can help regulate blood pressure. The warm flavor of the pumpkin contrasts beautifully with refreshing mango and dark red, antioxidant-rich hibiscus. The red pigments in hibiscus detox your heart.

Hibiscus Pumpkin Soup
WITH MANGO SALSA

Heat the butter in a large stockpot over medium heat. Add the onion and salt and cook, stirring occasionally, for 5 to 6 minutes, or until the onion starts to soften. Add the pumpkin puree and stock, stir to combine, and cook for 10 minutes more to allow the flavors to meld.

While the soup is cooking, prepare the hibiscus drizzle. Bring 1 cup of water to a boil in a small saucepan along with the honey. Add the hibiscus flowers or tea bags. Cook for 15 to 20 minutes, or until it reduces by half and forms a syrup.

To make the salsa, place the mango, cilantro, jalapeño, and vinegar in a bowl and toss well.

To serve, divide the soup among four bowls, drizzle each with the hibiscus syrup, and top with the mango salsa.

SERVES 4

2 tablespoons unsalted grass-fed butter or olive oil

½ medium-size onion, minced

½ teaspoon salt

1 (15-ounce) can pure pumpkin puree

1 quart vegetable stock

HIBISCUS DRIZZLE

½ cup dried hibiscus flowers, or 4 hibiscus tea bags

2 tablespoons honey or agave nectar

MANGO SALSA

1 small mango, peeled and cubed, or 1 cup frozen mango cubes, thawed

½ cup chopped fresh cilantro

1 jalapeño pepper, thinly sliced

1 tablespoon balsamic vinegar

per serving
192 calories
7 g (4 g) fat (sat)
30 g carbs
13 g sugar
4 g fiber
2 g protein
633 mg sodium

127

CONJUNCTION

Variety is one of the easiest ways to make your meals more pleasurable, and this is a far cry from the same old steamed broccoli. Harissa is an African chili paste that adds a kick, but you can also use sriracha or your standard jarred tomato salsa. Synonymous with love and the heart, rose petals add crunch and beauty, and make this dish a sensual pleasure to behold.

Roasted Broccoli
WITH HARISSA, CLOVES, AND ROSE

SERVES 4

2 tablespoons olive oil

1 head broccoli, cut into florets

¼ teaspoon salt

⅛ teaspoon ground cloves

1 tablespoon harissa or tomato paste

¼ cup shredded soft farmer cheese, mozzarella, or coconut cream

2 tablespoons food-grade rose petals or sesame seeds

Heat 1 tablespoon of the olive oil in a large, ovenproof skillet over medium heat. Add the broccoli, salt, and cloves, cover, and cook, turning occasionally, for 10 to 15 minutes, or until the broccoli is browned and tender. Place the harissa in a small bowl along with the remaining tablespoon of olive oil and stir well to combine. Dot the harissa sauce over the broccoli. If using cheese, sprinkle the cheese over the broccoli and place under the broiler for 1 to 2 minutes to melt. If using the coconut cream, spoon it over the broccoli as soon as it is browned and tender and skip the broiler step. Sprinkle with the rose petals. Serve immediately.

per serving
186 calories
12 g (4 g) fat (sat)
17 g carbs
11 g sugar
3 g fiber
3 g protein
215 mg sodium

THE SUPERFOOD ALCHEMY COOKBOOK

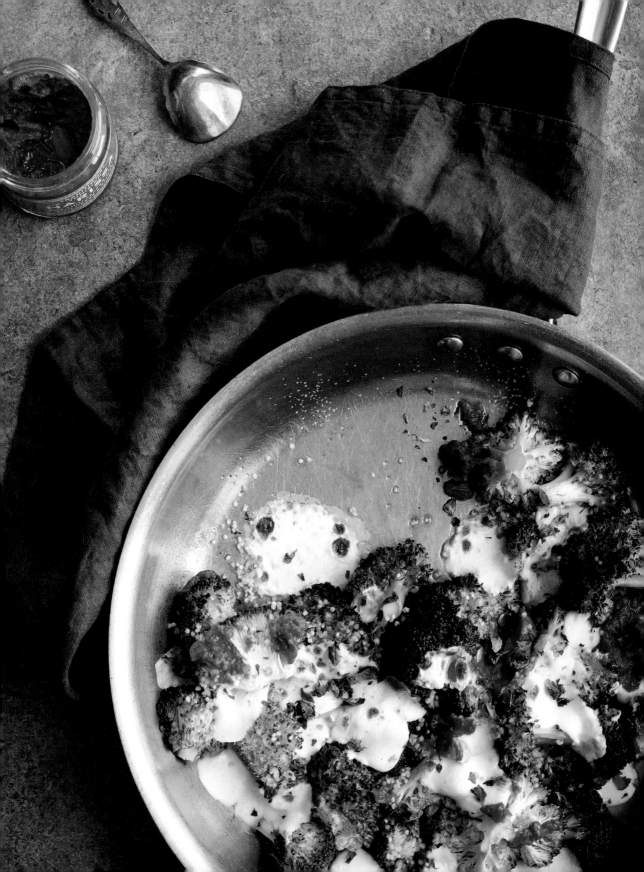

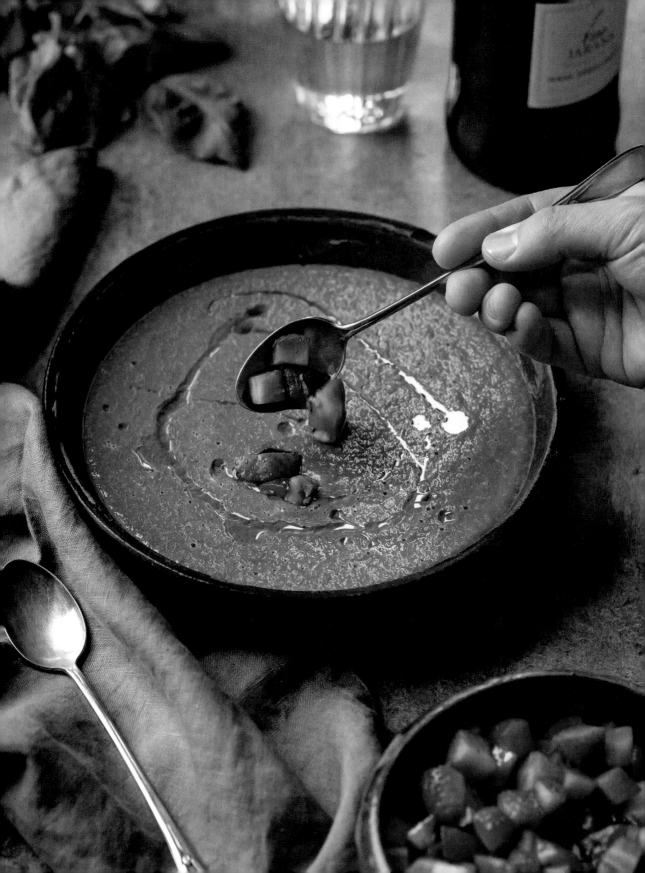

Basil and spinach are a healing pair for the heart, since basil contains compounds that relax your arteries, while the antioxidants in spinach help protect your blood and organ tissue. When time is scarce or fatigue sets in after work, turn to nourishing no-cook recipes like this one; simple, low-stress meal preparation is a great way to practice loving self-care.

Silky Basil Spinach Soup
WITH STRAWBERRY BALSAMIC SALSA

SERVES 4

To make the strawberry balsamic salsa, place the strawberries in a medium-size bowl along with the vinegar, 2 tablespoons of the olive oil, and ¼ cup of the basil. Toss well and set aside to let the flavors meld while you prepare the soup.

Place the remaining ¾ cup of basil and the spinach, stock or tea, scallions, cucumber, celery, avocado, hemp seeds, garlic, salt, and pepper in a high-speed blender. Puree until smooth. Divide among four bowls. Drizzle with the remaining tablespoon of olive oil and serve immediately topped with the salsa.

1 quart strawberries, hulled and sliced

¼ cup balsamic vinegar

3 tablespoons olive oil

1 cup fresh basil, sliced

1 pound spinach

2 cups vegetable stock or brewed green tea

2 scallions, quartered

½ medium-size cucumber, sliced

1 celery stalk, quartered

½ avocado, pitted and peeled

¼ cup hemp seeds, cashews, or almonds

½ medium-size garlic clove

½ teaspoon salt

¼ teaspoon freshly ground black pepper

per serving
382 *calories*
20 g (3 g) *fat (sat)*
23 g *carbs*
11 g *sugar*
8 g *fiber*
9 g *protein*
545 mg *sodium*

131

Great for gut health but also for your heart since they are packed with fiber, apples make a wonderfully sweet counterpoint to the salty tamari in this tasty Korean BBQ sauce. If your local grocer is short on portobellos, use their "baby" counterparts, Cremini mushrooms.

Korean BBQ Broccoli
WITH PORTOBELLOS AND FRIED SHALLOTS

SERVES 4

SAUCE

1 apple, cored, peeled, and cubed

2 to 3 garlic cloves, crushed

1 (1-inch) piece ginger, peeled

3 tablespoons low-sodium tamari

1 tablespoon honey or agave nectar, or 1 teaspoon stevia

1 tablespoon cornstarch

3 tablespoons sesame oil

1 head broccoli, roughly chopped

2 large portobello mushroom caps (about 8 ounces)

Cooking spray

3 shallots, thinly sliced

1 teaspoon sesame seeds

¼ teaspoon freshly ground black pepper

To make the sauce: Place the apple, garlic, and ginger in a food processor and finely chop. Add the tamari, honey or agave, and cornstarch along with 2 tablespoons of water and process until a chunky mixture forms. Set aside.

Remove the dark gills from under the mushrooms, using a spoon. Discard the gills and thinly slice the mushrooms.

Heat the sesame oil in a large skillet, preferably cast iron, over medium heat. Add the broccoli and the mushrooms and cook for 8 to 10 minutes, or until the mushrooms give off their liquid and the broccoli is tender. Lower the heat and add the sauce, tossing well to coat.

Cover and cook for 1 minute more until sauce thickens.

Coat a small skillet with cooking spray and heat over medium heat. Add the shallot and cook until crisp, 7 to 8 minutes, stirring occasionally. Sprinkle over the broccoli mushroom mixture. Serve immediately, sprinkled with the sesame seeds and pepper.

per serving

202 *calories*

11 g (2 g) *fat (sat)*

24 g *carbs*

13 g *sugar*

5 g *fiber*

6 g *protein*

801 mg *sodium*

This platter layers two heart-healthy foods, cauliflower and beans, with tempting nacho toppings. Cauliflower, like all cruciferous vegetables, contain sulforaphane and other nutrients, including vitamin C and potassium, which help regulate a healthy heart. Black beans are a humble superfood bursting with cholesterol-lowering fiber, and they also contain an extremely high level of antioxidants, like you'll find in blueberries.

Queso Cauliflower Nacho Platter
WITH CHIPOTLE TOMATO SALSA

Preheat to oven to 400°F and line a baking sheet with parchment paper. Place the tomatoes and garlic on the prepared baking sheet and roast for 20 to 25 minutes, or until the tomatoes start to brown. Transfer to a plate to cool. Once cool, place in a food processor along with the chipotle, lime zest and juice, and salt and process to your desired texture. Stir in the onion.

To rice the cauliflower, place the florets in a food processor and roughly chop. You will need to do this in two or three batches. Spread out the tortilla chips onto the parchment-covered baking sheet where you roasted the tomatoes. Sprinkle with the beans and top with the cauli-flower rice. Dot with half the salsa and sprinkle with the two types of cheese. Bake for 20 to 25 minutes, or until the cheese melts. Serve immediately with the remaining salsa.

SERVES 6

3 tomatoes (about 1 pound)

1 garlic clove

2 tablespoon chopped chipotle chile

Zest and juice of 1 lime

¼ teaspoon salt

2 tablespoons minced red onion

1 head cauliflower, cut into florets

1 (10-ounce) bag corn tortilla chips

1 (15-ounce) can black beans, drained and well rinsed

1 cup crumbled feta cheese or crumbled firm tofu

1 cup grated farmer white cheese or shredded vegan cheese

---
per serving
483 calories
22 g (9 g) fat (sat)
54 g carbs
8 g sugar
9 g fiber
18 g protein
744 mg sodium

133

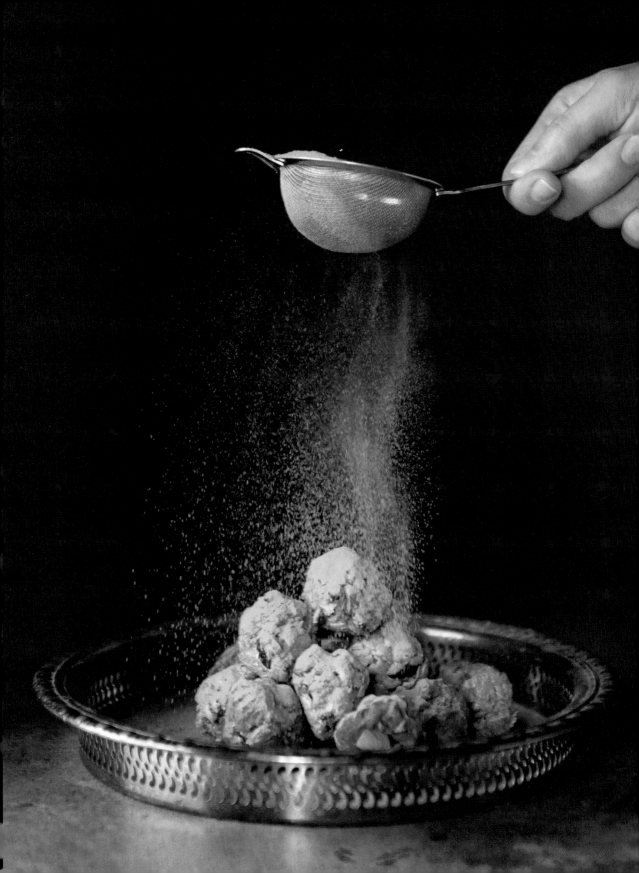

Grab a couple of these bites instead of that packaged protein bar postworkout and you'll be noshing on heart-healthy ingredients. Almonds, used here in both whole and nut butter form, are rich in folate, mono- and polyunsaturated fatty acids, and polyphenols— all nutrients that can soothe a stressed-out ticker. Cacao nibs, 100 percent real cacao, adds awesome crunch and chocolaty flavor, making these a nutritious swap for desserts as well, and contain flavonols that may improve blood flow, oxygen levels, and nerve function.

ALMOND CHOCOLATE CRUNCH
Protein Bites

Combine all the ingredients, except the turmeric or cocoa powder, in a medium-size mixing bowl and stir until evenly mixed. With clean hands, roll into balls about the size of a walnut, dust with the turmeric (if using), and refrigerate to set.

Store at room temperature or refrigerate.

NOTE: For a flavor twist, add 2 tablespoons of chopped dried cherries and ½ teaspoon of almond extract.

**MAKES 36 BITES
(18 SERVINGS)**

1 cup rolled oats

½ cup vanilla protein powder

½ cup creamy almond butter

¼ cup honey or stevia

¼ cup salted almonds, chopped

¼ cup cacao nibs

1 teaspoon pure vanilla extract

1 teaspoon turmeric or unsweetened cocoa powder, for dusting (optional)

2 bites with honey		*2 bites with stevia*	
110	*calories*	**96**	*calories*
7 g (1 g)	*fat (sat)*	**7 g (1 g)**	*fat (sat)*
10 g	*carbs*	**9 g**	*carbs*
5 g	*sugar*	**2 g**	*sugar*
2 g	*fiber*	**2 g**	*fiber*
4 g	*protein*	**4 g**	*protein*
29 mg	*sodium*	**28 mg**	*sodium*

135

This is a gluten-free version of the famous French pastry. The hibiscus-infused syrup adds an irresistible floral sweetness as well as healthy metabolic benefits. Most financier pans or molds make rectangular pastries. However, you can get creative and choose fun shaped molds to bake your financiers in—just watch them carefully, as smaller shapes may bake faster.

Almond Financiers
WITH HIBISCUS SYRUP

**MAKES 24 FINANCIERS
(24 SERVINGS)**

6 tablespoons unsalted grass-fed butter or vegan butter spread

¼ cup dried hibiscus flowers

2 tablespoons honey or agave syrup

Olive oil cooking spray

1 cup finely ground almonds

⅔ cup powdered sugar, plus 2 tablespoons more for garnish (optional)

¼ cup ground flax meal

Pinch of salt

Place the butter in a small saucepan and melt on low heat, about 3 minutes. Set aside to cool.

To make the hibiscus syrup, place the hibiscus flowers in 1 cup of water and bring to a boil. Cook for 10 to 15 minutes, or until a dark red liquid forms and reduces by one third. Strain to remove the flowers and discard them. Whisk the honey into the reduced liquid.

Preheat the oven to 350°F. Coat a mini-muffin or madeleine pan with the cooking spray. In a large bowl, combine the almonds, powdered sugar, flax, and salt. Stir to blend. Add ¼ cup of water-room temperature and mix until thoroughly blended. Add the melted butter and mix until thoroughly blended. The mixture will be gooey.

Spoon the batter into the molds, filling them about halfway to the rim. Drizzle with the hibiscus syrup. Place the baking sheet in the center of the oven and bake for 15 to 20 minutes, or until the edges of the financiers start to brown but the centers are still soft. Remove the baking sheet from the oven and let the financiers cool in the molds for 10 minutes. Unmold and let cool completely on racks or on parchment. If you like, dust the financiers with the additional powdered sugar before serving.

— ◇ —
per serving
81 *calories*
6 g (2 g) *fat (sat)*
7 g *carbs*
5 g *sugar*
1 g *fiber*
2 g *protein*
12 mg *sodium*
— ◇ —

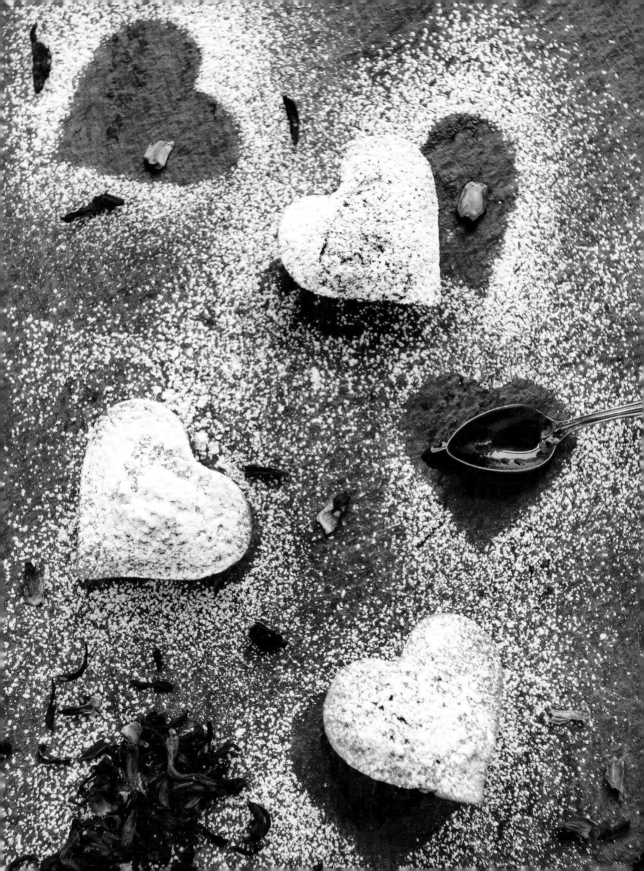

Heartburn is typically caused by a mixture of stress and not enough hydrochloric acid in the stomach. Low hydrochloric acid can slow digestion and cause the opening from the stomach to the esophagus to open up, which allows acid to come up the throat. This drinkable homemade cure is a great remedy—as is meditation. Try decreasing your consumption of foods that can be heartburn triggers, such as red wine, coffee, citrus, and vinegar.

Heartburn Cure

SERVES 1

1 (3-inch) piece fresh ginger
¼ teaspoon ground turmeric

Wash the ginger well under cold water. Rough chop it by hand or in a food processor. Place in a small saucepan with 2 cups of water and bring to a simmer over medium heat. Cook for 3 to 4 minutes, or until heated through. Stir in the turmeric and serve immediately.

2 cups	
16	calories
0 g (0 g)	fat (sat)
4 g	carbs
0 g	sugar
0 g	fiber
0 g	protein
3 mg	sodium

THE SUPERFOOD ALCHEMY COOKBOOK

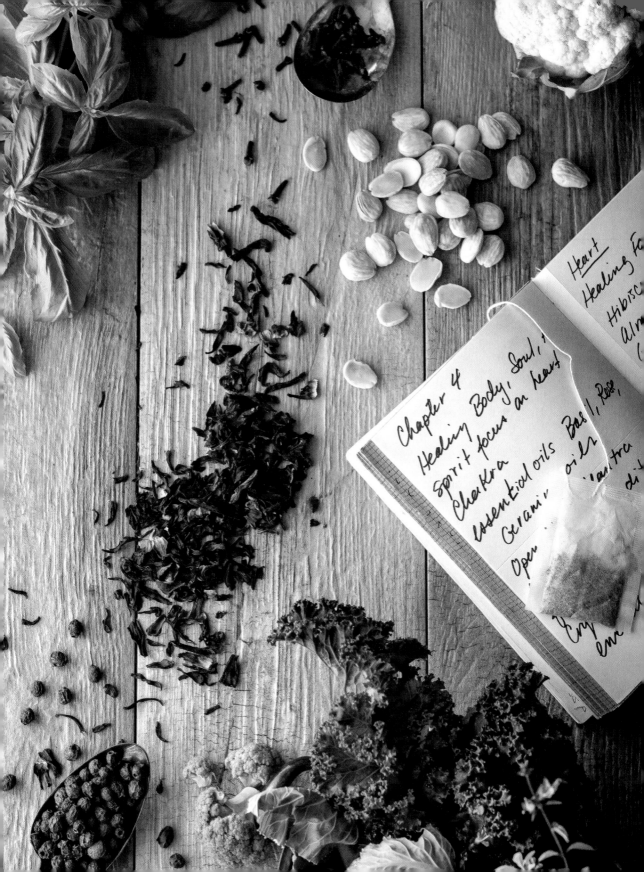

Essential Oil Preparations and Rituals for Conjunction

DIFFUSER OIL BLEND FOR ROMANTIC PASSION

Rose is a powerful flower scent that can be too strong or cloying for many people. Mixing it with spicy, earthy black pepper melds it into a seductive scent that's not overly floral and very intriguing.

4 drops black pepper essential oil

2 drops rose essential oil

Fill your essential oil diffuser with water according to the diffuser instructions. Add the oils and turn on the mister.

DIFFUSER OIL BLEND FOR EASING HEARTACHE

Use this fresh blend, with a hint of celery, to remind yourself that new experiences, friendships, and loves are just a matter of bringing fresh energy into your life.

2 to 3 drops angelica root essential oil

2 drops geranium essential oil

Fill your essential oil diffuser with water according to the diffuser instructions. Add the oils and turn on the mister.

SOLID PERFUME

If you want to be close and confident in the presence of your beloved, a little scent can make you feel fresh with a hint of romance. A petite dose of sweet perfume is the perfect, leakproof addition to any purse or gym bag. This mix isn't overly floral but if you enjoy floral scents you can increase the rose essential oil by one drop while decreasing the cardamom by one drop.

MAKES 2 LIP BALMS

2 (10 ml) lip balm containers

1 tablespoon coconut oil

1 teaspoon beeswax

3 drops sandalwood essential oil

2 drops cardamom essential oil

1 drop rose essential oil

Open the lip balm containers and place them on the countertop. Place the coconut oil and beeswax in a small saucepan over very low heat. Heat for 1 to 2 minutes, or until the wax melts completely. Turn off the heat. Add the essential oils and stir. Transfer to a measuring cup with a spout and pour the liquid into the lip balm containers. Let cool, then cap. Use to dab onto neck and pulse points.

VAPOR CHEST RUB

This chest rub with help open stuffed nasal passages and ease that congested feeling in your chest when you have a cold. Eucalyptus's anti-inflammatory compounds may trigger immune response, according to some small studies, making it a helpful partner in cold recovery.

MAKES ABOUT 1 CUP

1 tablespoon beeswax

1 cup coconut oil

10 drops eucalyptus essential oil

10 drops peppermint essential oil

5 drops geranium essential oil

Place the beeswax and coconut oil in a small saucepan over very low heat. Heat for 1 to 2 minutes, or until the wax melts completely. Turn off the heat. Add the essential oils and stir. Store in a small airtight container and use to rub over your chest when you are congested.

NOTE: One random study on eucalyptus oil used as aromatherapy after knee replacement surgery showed that pain in participants decreased just after participants in the study sniffed the oil.

Dry Brushing

Dry brushing is an exfoliating technique using a brush made from natural materials to brush your skin, to remove dryness, and to improve circulation. This practice, also said to stimulate the lymphatic system, is at the core of all its benefits. For a simple dry brushing practice, start at your feet and hands and brush up your legs and arms, brushing toward your heart center. Brush your entire body, except your face, continuing to brush in the direction of your heart, applying gentle pressure. You can incorporate essential oils into your dry brushing by adding a few drops of oil that you tolerate well directly to the bristles, or using one of the lotions or massage oil blends from this book.

Healing Stone Therapy
Rose quartz, emerald, and chrysoprase are all healing crystals for this area. While practicing any of the meditations featured in this book, you can rest one of these crystals on the center of your breastbone. To be more open hearted or to help heal heartache, wear one of these crystals on a longer necklace, allowing the stone to touch the center of your breastbone.

Quick Heart Energy Center Adjustment

Have you ever heard the expression "You wear your heart on your sleeve," meaning that your feelings are really visible to others? Body language and specifically posture can also tell you a lot about the balance of emotions, body, and mind. Posture can also be reliable way to recognize when an energy center needs emotional and psychological therapy, so check yourself out in the mirror or have a friend take a photo from time to time when you're not expecting it, to see how you're holding yourself. We tend to slouch in areas of the body where there is weakness; we hunch over and close down areas where we've been injured, or where we have negative feelings. Rounded shoulders can be a sign you're carrying negative energies in your heart energy center. Try this easy mind-body tweak to open the heart area. Place a small throw pillow or yoga block on the floor. Sit in front of the pillow or block, positioning yourself so that when you lie down, the pillow or block will be at the center of your back behind the heart area. Lie back with your arms extended to either side, looking at the ceiling, to allow the chest to open as you rest for at least 5 minutes. Alternatively, if you own a foam roller, sit on one end of the roller (or the floor if you are very tall), and line up the roller parallel with your spine. Lie across the roller so your head is also supported, opening your arms to either side, resting the back of your palms on the floor. Repeat several times a week or combine with any of the meditations in this book, or an essential oil diffuser blend.

Conjunction Meditation

In alchemy, feminine and masculine energies are associated with opposite ideas or principles. Feminine is associated with feelings, receiving, right-brain activities such as creativity and intuition, and "being." Masculine is associated with thinking, giving, and taking action or "doing." Conjunction is the coming together of the feminine and masculine energies inside you by balancing emotions and thoughts to become more intuitive and honest about who you are. Energy inside the body (the same energy that you feel from our sex organs) can be harnessed and use in a more thoughtful way. By using both hemispheres of the brain, creativity and logic, in a more sophisticated way instead of just for raw sex or feeding physical desires, your passion is channeled into work that is more transformative. This creates a sense of "solidness" or groundedness, and the feeling of "being on the right track and living up to our own potential," which is why the element earth is associate with this alchemical operation.

Find a comfortable seat. Choose a soothing song to play during your meditation. Close your eyes and begin to breathe deeply through your nose. Feel your belly rise and fall as if you are initiating the breath from your stomach. Continue to breathe from your stomach, expanding it first, and slowing down the breath to a count of four. Clear your thoughts and start to feel the energy around your sex organs, a tingling sensation. Ignore any thoughts of fear, shame, or sexual fantasies, or memories; just feel the energy. Visualize it as a match striking and catching fire. Allow that energy to build heat in your body and creep up into your belly, feel it start to rise, like mercury in a thermometer on a hot day. Allow it to continue to rise toward your belly button. Now, mentally focus on your job (if it's your life's purpose) or your dream job even if you think it's out of your reach. Imagine that you are doing activities around this work, whatever the activities are, and that you are doing them well. Hold onto these thoughts as you reconnect with the heat energy rising through your body, in the direction of your heart. Once the energy hits the heart center, exhale and rest there, clearing your mind once again of thoughts. When the music ends you can slowly open your eyes, slowly moving your hands and feet. Gently rotate your head around to release the neck. Slowly rise and resume your day.

Bare Your Heart Ritual

Want more love energy to flow? Try this easy ritual can help get love energy flow from your heart and bring your loved ones closer to you as well. One of the biggest regrets people report, when loved ones pass, is not telling them how they felt about them.

To begin purchase a beautiful card or piece of stationary. Anoint the paper with a drop of any of the essential oils from this chapter. Write a few simple lines telling your loved one how you feel or even why you are grateful for, and specifically something that is difficult for your to verbalize. Don't forget to post it!

143

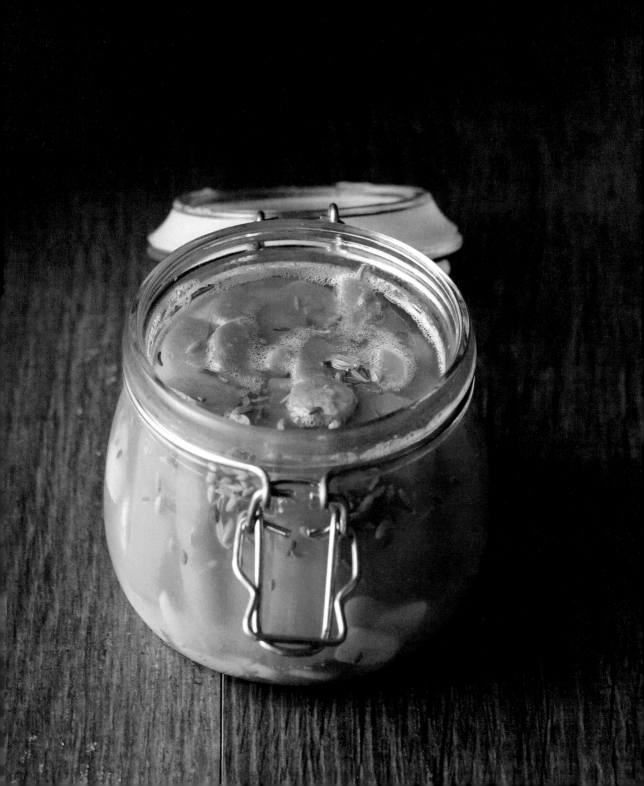

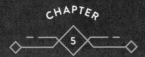

CHAPTER

5

Fermentation

SPEAKING YOUR TRUTH AND PROTECTING THE THYROID

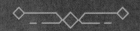

Fermentation is commonly associated with gut health, but the process is also tied to this energy center.

If you feel that the daily activities of life have left you feeling a bit lackluster, this throat-centric energy center is a great place to work. The recipes and therapies in this chapter correspond to the area surrounding the thyroid, a butterfly-shape gland situated low on the front of the neck, below the Adam's apple. This area is associated with self-expression and communication, and the alchemical process of fermentation.

Fermentation is commonly associated with gut health, but the process is also tied to this energy center. The processes of fermentation and digestion are interrelated, and digestion doesn't only happen in the gut! That is one of the reasons the area around the mouth and throat is a focus here: digestion actually starts when we chew and enzymes in the mouth start to break down our food. Similarly, when we make fermented food, such as the pickles on page 162, the vegetables begin to break down and are partially digested by the helpful invisible microbes called lactobacillus, which also happen to be very healthy for our gut. Pickles start out as bland vegetables and are then, somewhat miraculous, turned into something far more sophisticated and tangy through fermentation.

Like the process of fermentation in food, fermentation in alchemy is the "dying" or shedding of the old and a revivification of the new. We discard old ways of thinking and living that no longer serve us, and begin to look at life with fresh perspective. This process can be totally transformative—just think of the difference between that bland cucumber and the zesty pickle. If you've gone through a major life change, you may understand this: once you pull through a "dying" phase, where you may have experienced loss, grief, and stress, you begin to experience life with a new excitement.

The thyroid gland controls your body temperature, heartbeat, and metabolism, along with many other functions that provide energy and strength throughout the body. Nearly every cell in the body needs thyroid hormones, so when the thyroid isn't functioning, a slew of symptoms can result. Genetics, nutritional deficiencies, environmental toxins, gluten sensitivity, and stress are all factors that can cause the thyroid to go haywire. Because stress and fatigue can play a role, the alchemical lesson for protecting your thyroid health is to slow down and just allow. Instead of working that extra hour or having that last drink, allow for peaceful alone time, regularly scheduled sleep, and enjoy the bounty of soulful essential oil recipes in this book.

Superfoods, Herbs, and Essential Oils for the Throat and Thyroid

SEAWEED: A great plant-based source of the essential nutrient iodine. The thyroid gland takes iodine from food and converts it into thyroid hormones thyroxine (T4) and triiodothyronine (T3). Every cell in the body depends on thyroid hormones, and thus needs iodine, to regulate metabolism.

BRAZIL NUTS: Selenium, a supernutrient that your thyroid needs to activate an enzyme that circulates T4 and T3, is found in incredibly high amounts in Brazil nuts. In fact, just noshing on two or three can provide you with your daily RDA for selenium. Limit yourself to four nuts per day.

ARTICHOKE: Traditionally considered to be both a medicinal and superfood for the liver, high-fiber artichokes have much to offer for overall health. Eating more high-fiber foods, including prebiotic foods, is linked to better sleep, a must for healthy thyroid function, since sleep deprivation hits the thyroid hard. Liver health and thyroid are deeply linked, as thyroid diseases are frequently associated with liver injuries.

CILANTRO: Also called Chinese parsley, cilantro may help the body to detox heavy metals when paired with other cleansing protocols. Heavy metals can be crippling for your thyroid when they bond with molecules present in T4 and T3 (for example, when mercury is stored in the thyroid in place of iodine).

CHAMOMILE AND CHAMOMILE ESSENTIAL OIL: Calming chamomile has long been an herbal remedy to help people "on the go" wind down, a must-have for A types or for those who just work too many hours. Getting adequate rest is one of the ways you can bolster thyroid health. The oil has many of the same healing compounds as the herb; the oil is actually blue in color due to the active organic compound azulene.

ASHWAGANDHA: An adaptogenic herb ground from the root of the plant, ashwagandha may be a way to give your thyroid a boost. Some studies show it can help normalize both underactive and overactive thyroid by triggering the serum thyroid stimulating hormone (TSH).

TEA TREE OIL: Native to Australia, the tea tree plant produces a strongly scented oil. Astringent, antiviral, and antibacterial, tea tree oil is an excellent remedy for sore throats and respiratory infections. Be warned: tea tree oil has a strongly medicinal flavor and is not to be consumed orally.

EUCALYPTUS OIL: Another Australian plant with a long list of therapeutic uses, eucalyptus oil is antibacterial, antimicrobial, and excellent for pain relief. It has a refreshing scent reminiscent of pine, mint, and honey.

In folk medicine traditions, eucalyptus is used as a remedy for cold sores as well as respiratory problems, perhaps due to its antibacterial and antimicrobial properties and its minty like odor that can help open nasal passages.

Ashwagandha has adaptogenic properties that can help reduce stress and anxiety, making it a perfect morning ritual to maintain calm throughout the day—one of the essential components of thyroid care! Like other berries, blackberries are rich in vitamin C and antioxidants.

Blackberry Vanilla Smoothie
WITH ASHWAGANDHA

SERVES 2

2 cups blackberries

⅔ cup protein powder or Greek yogurt

1 cup grass-fed dairy milk or coconut milk

1 tablespoon honey or agave nectar

2 teaspoons powdered ashwagandha

1 teaspoon pure vanilla extract

8 ice cubes

Place the blackberries, protein powder or Greek yogurt, milk, honey, ashwagandha, vanilla, and ice cubes in a blender. Process until smooth. Divide between two cups and serve immediately.

per serving	
239	calories
5 g (3 g)	fat (sat)
32 g	carbs
20 g	sugar
11 g	fiber
20 g	protein
104 mg	sodium

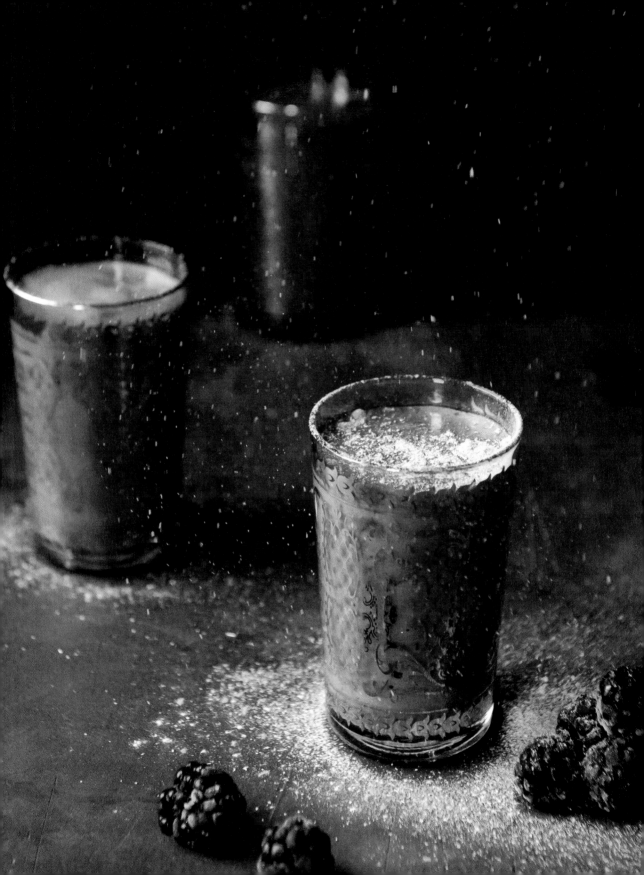

This creamy smoothie gets its texture from antioxidant-packed mangoes and joint-healthy coconut milk. Its heaping serving of spirulina adds phytonutrients that help protect against free radicals and provide an easy way to squeeze in the thyroid-boosting nutrient iodine. Brazil nuts are a superfood, but limit yourself to four nuts per day.

MANGO
Spirulina Smoothie

SERVES 2

2 cup fresh or frozen mango

2 cups baby spinach

⅔ cup protein powder or Greek yogurt

1 cup grass-fed dairy milk or coconut milk

¼ cup Brazil nuts

2 teaspoons powdered spirulina

8 ice cubes

Place the mango, spinach, protein powder, milk, Brazil nuts, spirulina, and ice cubes in a blender. Process until smooth. Divide between two cups and serve immediately.

1½ cups	*cups*
360	*calories*
16 g (6 g)	*fat (sat)*
38 g	*carbs*
28 g	*sugar*
8 g	*fiber*
24 g	*protein*
159 mg	*sodium*

The yogurt in this probiotic Mediterranean-inspired dressing contains beneficial bacteria to aid digestion. The dressing is similar to tzatziki, and any leftover sauce makes a great dipping condiment for cut veggies. Feel free to incorporate any other fresh herbs, such as dill or mint, to add an extra layer of flavor.

Cleansing Spring Salad
WITH YOGURT DRESSING

SERVES 4

Cook the millet according to the package instructions. Set aside.

Prepare the dressing: Place ¼ cup of water and the yogurt, chives, pickle, cilantro or parsley, shallot, mayonnaise, mustard, vinegar, salt, and pepper in a large bowl. Whisk until smooth.

Arrange the watercress, artichokes, cucumber, and radishes on a large platter. Sprinkle with the grains and drizzle with the dressing. Serve immediately.

½ cup uncooked millet or quinoa

DRESSING

½ cup whole-milk Greek yogurt or coconut yogurt

¼ cup chopped chives, or 2 green onions, chopped

¼ cup chopped bread-and-butter or dill pickle

¼ cup fresh cilantro or parsley, minced

1 small shallot, minced

¼ cup mayonnaise or vegan mayonnaise

1 teaspoon Dijon mustard

1 teaspoon raw cider vinegar

½ teaspoon salt

¼ teaspoon freshly ground black pepper

½ pound watercress

1 (9-ounce) package frozen artichoke hearts, defrosted, or 1 (15-ounce) can artichoke hearts, drained

1 large cucumber, thinly sliced or cubed

½ pound radishes, thinly sliced

—————◇—————
3 cups	
366	calories
23 g (4 g)	fat (sat)
30 g	carbs
7 g	sugar
8 g	fiber
9 g	protein
705 mg	sodium

—————◇—————

Salsa verde ("green salsa") is a refreshing Mexican condiment made with tomatillos and cilantro. If you've never tried a tomatillo, it's a nightshade fruit that is much less sweet than a tomato. Search for them in organic markets or any specialty shops that sell Latin groceries. Salsa verde also makes a great dipping sauce for a healthier spin on chips and dip—use your favorite raw or roasted veggies in place of chips.

SALSA VERDE
Cauliflower Rice Skillet

SERVES 4

2 medium-size heads cauliflower, cut into florets (about 2 pounds or 8 cups)

½ pound tomatillos

2 jalapeño peppers or 1 poblano pepper, seeded and diced

2 tablespoons minced red onion

Zest and juice of 1 lime

½ teaspoon salt

¼ teaspoon freshly ground black pepper

2 tablespoons unsalted grass-fed butter or coconut oil

1 tablespoon of olive oil

½ cup fresh cilantro, roughly chopped

½ shallot, minced

1 (15-ounce) can chickpeas or kidney beans, drained and rinsed

Preheat the oven to 400°F. To rice the cauliflower, place the florets in a food processor and roughly chop. You will need to do this in two or three batches. Set aside and prepare the salsa verde.

Remove and discard the husks from the tomatillos, and score the bottom of them making an X with a sharp paring knife. Place them on a baking sheet and roast for 15 to 20 minutes, or until the skins become golden. Remove from the oven and let them cool, about 15 minutes, then peel off the skins. Combine the peeled tomatillos, jalapeños, red onion, lime zest and juice, salt, and pepper in a food processor and pulse until thoroughly incorporated. Set aside.

Heat the butter or coconut oil and olive oil in a large skillet over medium heat. Add the cilantro and shallot and cook until softened, about 1 minute. Add the cauliflower rice and chickpeas and cook until heated through, about 2 minutes for al dente cauliflower, or up to 4 minutes for more tender cauliflower. Serve the cauliflower rice with the salsa verde.

ADDITIONAL NOTE: Cauliflower is not only bursting with vitamin C and cancer-preventative compounds, but it's also ideal for weight management after a weekend splurge.

per serving with butter 2 cups

250	calories
12 g (5 g)	fat (sat)
30 g	carbs
4g	sugar
10 g	fiber
10 g	protein
358 mg	sodium

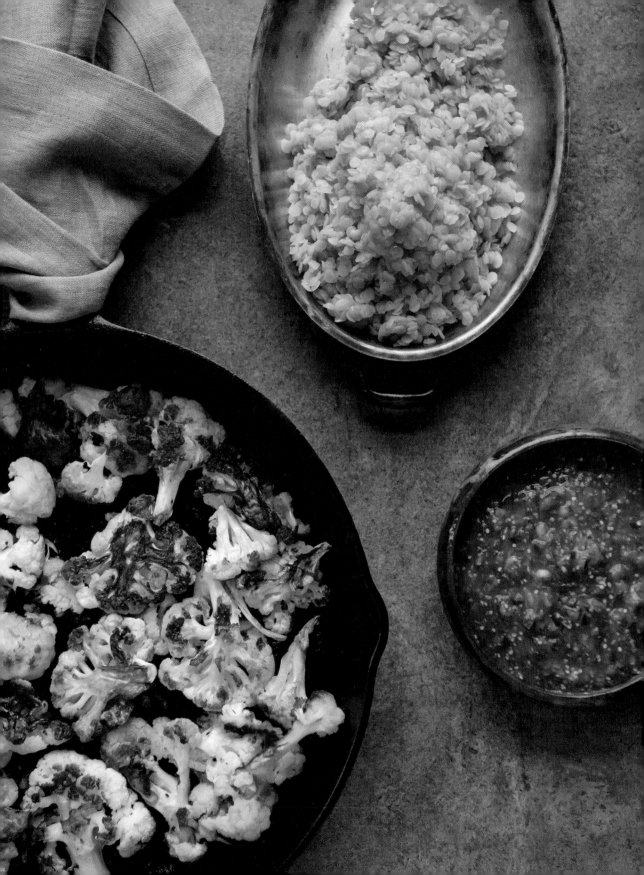

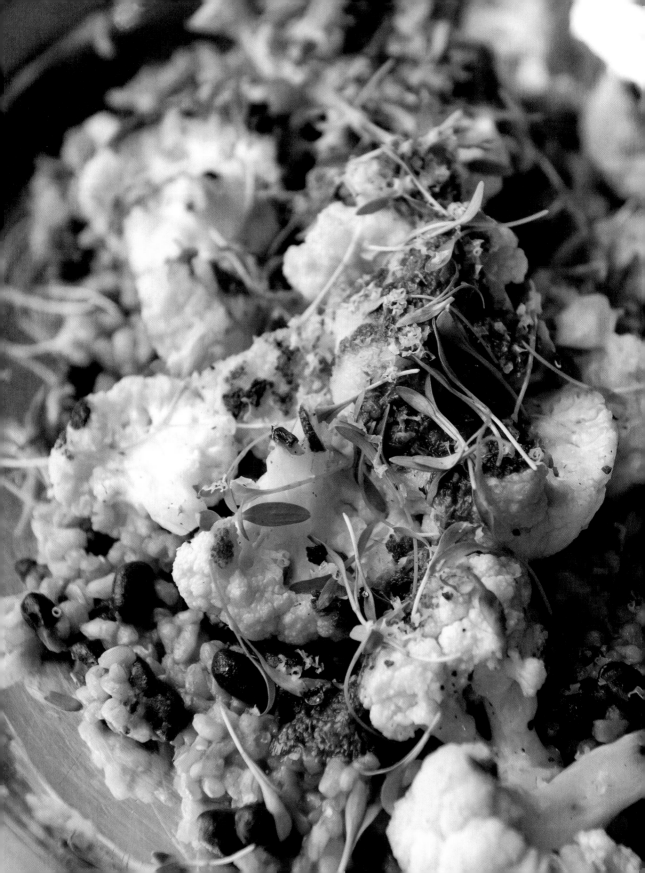

This rice and beans recipe is not only chock-full of healing superfoods, but it makes a hearty platter suitable for entertaining or make-ahead meals for the week. If you have leftovers, this platter heats up well and makes a killer office lunch—recipes that let you cook once and eat twice are great ways to free up your time and avoid stress.

CHIMICHURRI CAULIFLOWER
Black Beans and Rice Platter

SERVES 6

Cook the rice according to the package instructions. Heat 1 tablespoon of the butter or olive oil and ¼ teaspoon of the salt in a large skillet over medium heat. Add the chipotle chile and toss well, then cook, stirring, for an additional minute, or until the chile is fragrant. Add the beans and cooked rice and stir to combine.

Heat the remaining tablespoon of butter in another large skillet and add the cauliflower florets and the remaining ¼ teaspoon of salt. Cook, covered, stirring often, for 4 to 5 minutes, or until the cauliflower starts to brown and give off its liquid and soften.

Prepare the chimichurri sauce: Place the parsley and cilantro in a food processor along with the garlic. Pulse four or five times to roughly chop. Add the olive oil and vinegar and process until smooth.

Transfer the rice and beans to a platter and top with the cauliflower. Drizzle with the chimichurri sauce. Using a Microplane, grate the Brazil nuts over the rice, garnish with microgreens or cilantro, and serve immediately.

1 cup uncooked short-grain brown rice

2 tablespoons unsalted grass-fed butter or olive oil

½ teaspoon salt

2 tablespoons chopped chipotle chile in adobo

1 (15-ounce) can black beans, drained and well rinsed

1 large head cauliflower, cut into florets (about 8 cups)

½ cup fresh parsley leaves

½ cup fresh cilantro leaves and stems

1 garlic clove

¼ cup olive oil

1 tablespoon cider vinegar

2 Brazil nuts

½ cup microgreens of your choice or chopped cilantro for garnish (optional)

◇
per serving
239 *calories*
15 g (4 g) *fat (sat)*
25 g *carbs*
3 g *sugar*
7 g *fiber*
7 g *protein*
518 mg *sodium*
◇

When you're craving a slice of pizza, reach instead for this classic marinara recipe that makes veggie noodles crave-worthy! This recipe serves eight for a plant-based Italian Sunday dinner or can easily be cut in half to serve four.

ZUCCHINI
Marinara Spaghetti
WITH SHAVED BRAZIL NUTS

SERVES 8

1 tablespoon olive oil

1 garlic clove, minced

½ red onion or 2 large shallots, minced

2 tablespoons tomato paste

1 teaspoon dried oregano

2 (28-ounce) cans whole peeled tomatoes

1 cup white wine

4 pounds zucchini (about 4 large zucchini)

¼ cup shaved Brazil nuts (limit 4 nuts per day), or ½ cup Parmesan cheese, grated

Cooking spray (optional)

Heat the olive oil in a medium-size saucepan, about 30 seconds. Add the garlic and onion or shallots and cook until soft and aromatic, about 1 minute. Add the tomato paste and oregano and cook, stirring often, for 1 minute more, or until the tomato paste becomes fragrant. Add the tomatoes and wine, bring to a boil, and then lower the heat to low to maintain a simmer. Continue to cook, uncovered, until the liquid has reduced by half, about 30 minutes.

Trim both ends of the zucchini and process them according to your spiralizer or vegetable noodle maker instructions. Serve the "noodles" raw with the marinara sauce and shaved Brazil nuts. Alternatively, to serve the noodles hot, coat a large skillet with cooking spray and heat over medium heat. Add the vegetable noodles and cook for 2 to 3 minutes, or until the noodles start to soften and give off some their liquid, before topping with marinara and shaved Brazil nuts.

per serving with zucchini and Parmesan

148	*calories*
4 g (1 g)	*fat (sat)*
18 g	*carbs*
12 g	*sugar*
4 g	*fiber*
7 g	*protein*
460 mg	*sodium*

THE SUPERFOOD ALCHEMY COOKBOOK

The Goddess in alchemy is "divine feminine" energy, associated with right-brain activity, intuition, art, and feeling. This energy also relates to verbally expressing your emotions and speaking your truth, a function of alchemical fermentation. This recipe highlights two of this chapter's featured ingredients, cilantro and artichokes, in a healthful salad with a creamy, lemony dressing.

Honor the Goddess Green Salad
WITH CILANTRO RANCH DRESSING

Place the cilantro, tahini, mayonnaise, coconut milk, scallions, lemon zest and juice, garlic salt, and stevia in a food processor and process until smooth. Divide the greens among four plates, and top with the avocado, tomatoes, olives, and artichoke hearts. Drizzle with the dressing, then sprinkle with the paprika. Serve immediately.

SERVES 4

⅓ cup chopped fresh cilantro

3 tablespoons well-stirred tahini

3 tablespoons mayonnaise or vegan mayonnaise

⅓ cup coconut milk

2 scallions, chopped

Zest and juice of 1 small lemon

1 teaspoon garlic salt

½ teaspoon stevia

5 ounces mixed greens, power greens, or baby spinach

1 avocado, pitted, peeled, and diced

2 tomatoes, diced

½ cup pitted black olives

1 (15-ounce) can quartered artichoke hearts, drained and well rinsed

½ teaspoon mild paprika

3 cups salad with
¼ cup dressing
280 calories
21 g (3 g) fat (sat)
22 g carbs
4 g sugar
9 g fiber
7 g protein
704 mg sodium

Fried rice is a delicious dish that can be made into a satisfying meal in itself depending upon what you put in it. This version is amped up with kimchi, a traditional fermented Korean delicacy of spicy pickled cabbage or other vegetables. Many varieties of kimchi are available, so feel free to experiment with different kinds, and add other veggies that you have in your fridge.

KIMCHI BRUSSELS SPROUT
Fried Rice

SERVES 4

1 cup uncooked short-grain brown rice

3 tablespoons sesame or coconut oil

1 pound Brussels sprouts, trimmed and cut in half

2 cups broccoli florets

1 cup fresh or frozen corn kernels (defrost if frozen)

1 cup kimchi, chopped (for homemade, see page 162, or use store-bought)

Seaweed chips, thinly sliced

½ cup chopped fresh cilantro

Cook the rice according to the package instructions and set aside. Heat 2 tablespoons of the sesame oil in a large skillet over medium heat. Add the Brussels sprouts and broccoli to the skillet, cut side down, and cook for 5 to 6 minutes, or until the sprouts start to brown. Turn them and cook for 5 to 6 minutes more, or until tender.

Push the Brussels sprouts to the side and add the remaining tablespoon of oil. Add the corn and rice and cook for 2 to 3 minutes without stirring, to allow the rice to brown. Mix the Brussels sprouts into the rice. Add the kimchi and toss well. Top with seaweed chips and the cilantro and serve.

per serving
368 *calories*
15 g (9 g) *fat (sat)*
58 g *carbs*
6 g *sugar*
10 g *fiber*
10 g *protein*
351 mg *sodium*

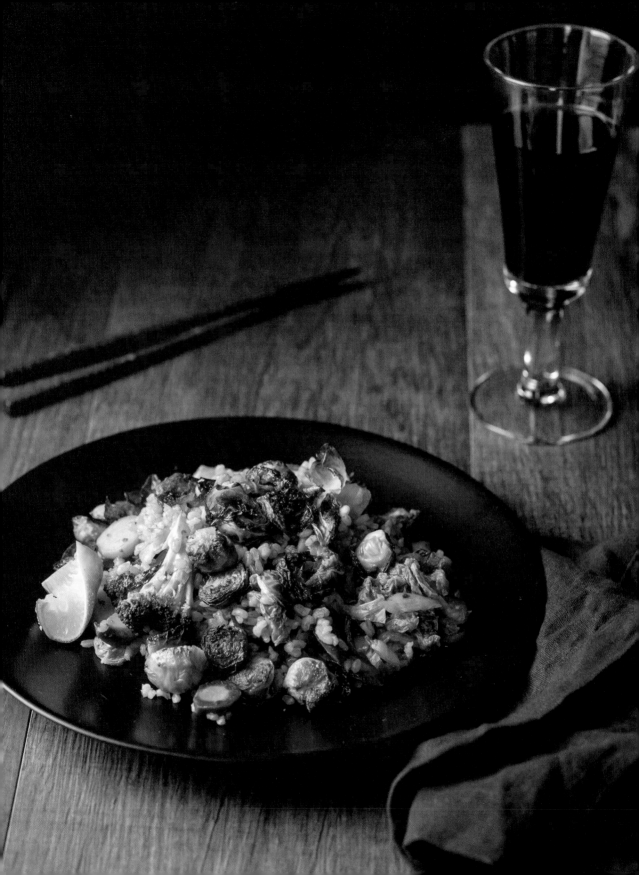

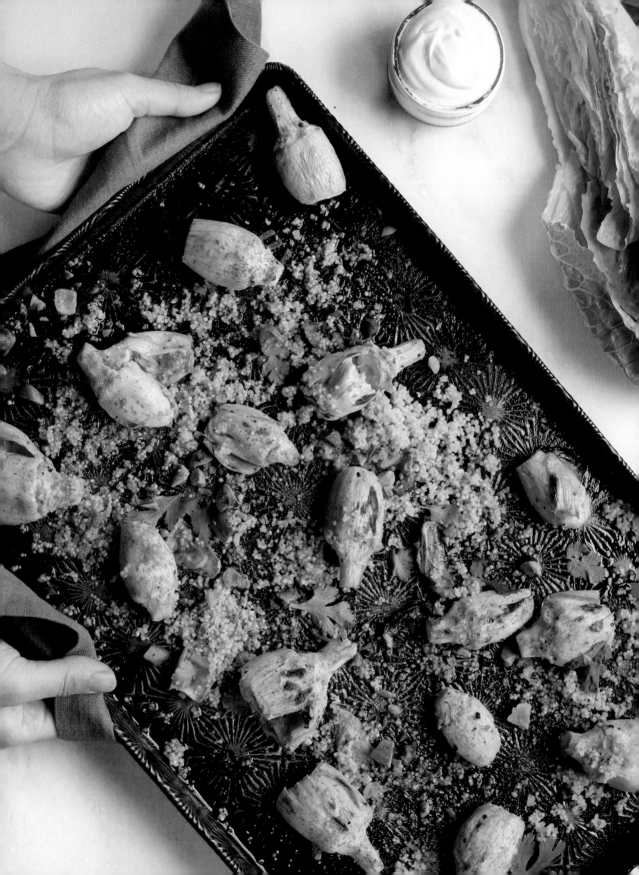

Artichokes come straight out of the can looking like beautiful pale roses, packed with flavor and nutrients. How amazing is that? This dish enhances the natural beauty of these vitamin-rich plants in the thistle family by baking them to a golden crisp and scattering them with crispy quinoa and pine nuts. This dish makes a wonderful appetizer; you can also serve it as a salad. Arrange 8 ounces of greens (such as baby spinach, kale, or mesclun mix) on your platter and top with the grains, artichokes, and lemon chamomile aioli before serving.

Roasted Artichoke Hearts
WITH LEMON CHAMOMILE AIOLI

Cook the quinoa according to the package instructions and set aside.

Preheat the oven to 400°F. Pat the artichoke hearts dry with a paper towel or dish towel. Place on a baking sheet and coat with a thin layer of cooking spray. Sprinkle with seasoning salt. Roast for 25 to 30 minutes, or until the artichokes start to brown.

Meanwhile, prepare the aioli: Place the mayonnaise in small bowl along with the lemon zest and juice, chamomile, and mustard and whisk well to combine.

Spread out the quinoa on a platter. Top with the artichokes, drizzle with the aioli, and garnish with cilantro and pine nuts or Brazil nuts. Serve immediately.

SERVES 4

½ cup uncooked quinoa or millet

2 (8.5-ounce) cans artichoke hearts, well drained

Olive oil cooking spray

½ teaspoon seasoning salt, such as Old Bay

⅓ cup olive oil–based mayonnaise or vegan mayonnaise

Zest and juice of 1 lemon

1½ tablespoon loose chamomile tea or crushed dried chamomile flowers, or the contents of 1 chamomile tea bag

¼ teaspoon Dijon mustard

¼ cup fresh cilantro leaves, torn

¼ cup pine nuts or chopped Brazil nuts

---◇---

per serving
284 calories
14 g (1 g) fat (sat)
34 g carbs
1 g sugar
14 g fiber
9 g protein
363 mg sodium

---◇---

These fermented vegetables can be used as garnish next to breakfast eggs, in a sandwich or salad, or as a component of a grain bowl. The ginger and turmeric make these pungent pickles powerful immune system strengtheners, and fermented dishes provide a healthy dose of probiotics.

Pickled Vegetable Trio:
KIMCHI, PICKLED CUCUMBERS, AND PICKLED CARROT

**SERVES 60; MAKES
4 QUARTS OF PICKLES**

1 (2-pound) napa cabbage

1 teaspoon salt

2 tablespoons harissa

*2 to 3 tablespoons
low-sodium tamari*

4 scallions, chopped

2 garlic cloves, minced

*2 tablespoons minced fresh
ginger*

*1 pound baby cucumbers,
such as Persian, quartered*

4 garlic cloves, thinly sliced

*1 (1-inch) piece fresh turmeric,
thinly sliced*

1 teaspoon cumin seeds

1 teaspoon coriander seeds

*1 pound carrots, peeled and
cut into thirds*

STEP 1 Remove the outer, rough damaged leaves of the cabbage. Rinse and chop into 2 by 2-inch pieces. Place in a large bowl along with ⅓ teaspoon of the salt. Squeeze the cabbage in the bowl, allowing some of the liquid to release. Toss with the harissa, tamari, scallions, garlic, and ginger.

STEP 2 Transfer the mixture to a 2-quart clamp-top jar and cover with enough water to submerge the cabbage, pressing it down under the water level, using a glass weight if necessary, to keep it submerged to prevent molding.

Place the cucumbers in large bowl with ⅓ teaspoon of the salt. Top with half of the sliced garlic cloves, the fresh turmeric, ½ teaspoon of the cumin seeds, and ½ teaspoon of the coriander seeds. Toss well. Repeat Step 2.

Bring a large pot of water to a boil and add the carrots. Cook for 4 to 5 minutes, or until the carrots are crisp-tender. Drain and cool slightly. Transfer the carrots to a large bowl along with the remaining ⅓ teaspoon of salt, garlic, cumin, and coriander seeds. Toss well. Repeat Step 2.

FERMENT at room temperature (60° to 70°F) for 3 to 4 days, or until the pickles reach your desired tanginess, then transfer to the fridge. Store, refrigerated, for up to 3 months.

*1 pickle, 2 carrots,
2 tablespoons kimchi*
9 *calories*
0 g (0 g) *fat (sat)*
2 g *carbs*
1 g *sugar*
1 g *fiber*
0 g *protein*
88 mg *sodium*

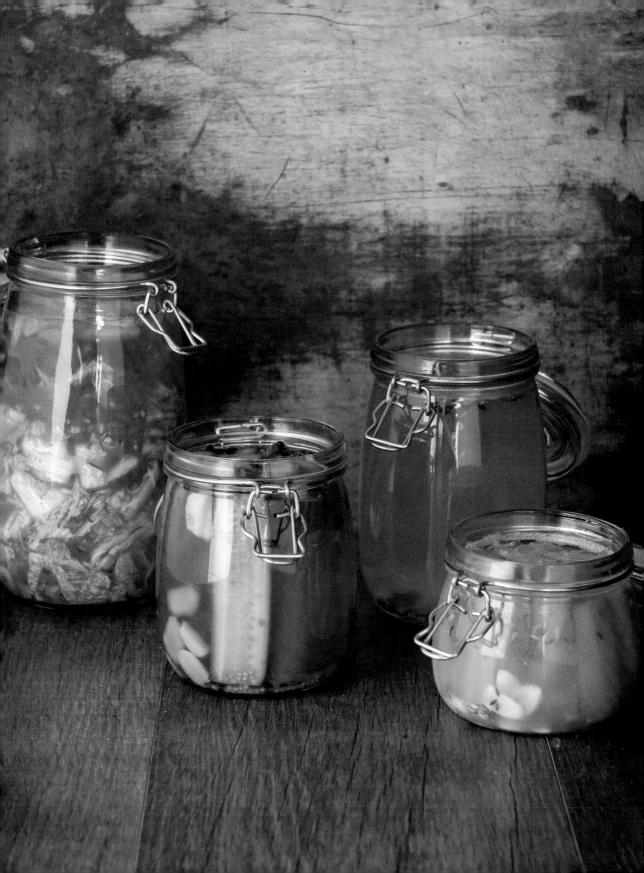

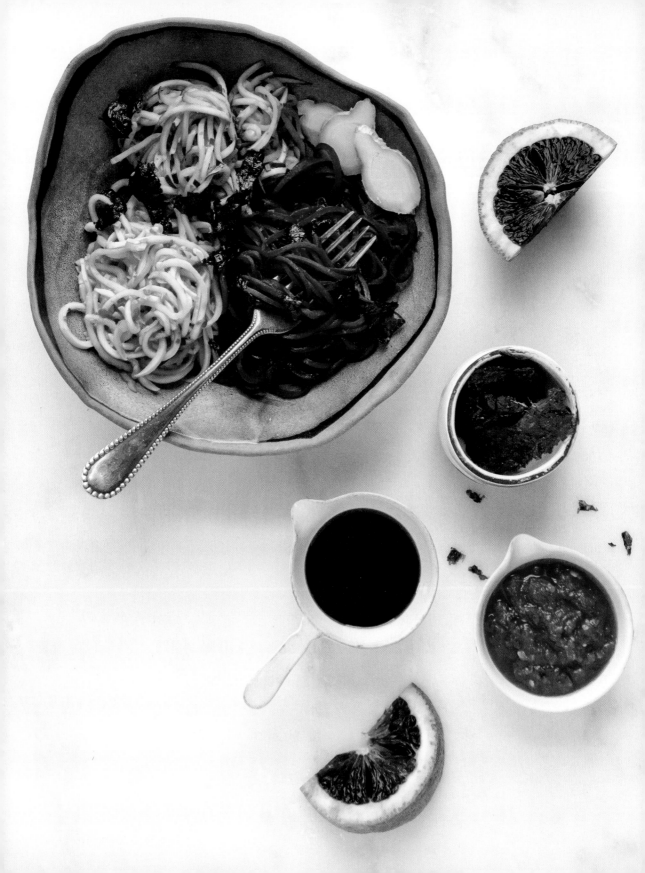

If you're craving a bowl of Asian noodles but want to skip the gluten bomb, try out this recipe, which will surely satisfy with its sweet and sour notes. Veggie noodles are an innovative way to get extra nutrients into your diet. You can serve any leftover sauce with broccoli for a tasty afternoon snack.

Orange Tamari Veggie Noodles
WITH CRISP SEAWEED

SERVES 4

Trim both ends of the squash and/or beets and process them according to your spiralizer or vegetable noodle maker instructions. Set aside.

To prepare the sauce, combine the scallions, orange zest and juice, tamari, honey or agave, vinegar, sesame oil, garlic, ginger, cornstarch, chili garlic sauce, and pepper in a small saucepan, whisking to remove any clumps of cornstarch. Bring to a simmer over medium heat to thicken the sauce, 4 to 5 minutes. Once the mixture thickens, remove the pan from heat.

Coat a large skillet with cooking spray and heat over medium heat. Add the vegetable noodles and cook for 2 to 3 minutes, or until the noodles start to soften and give off some their liquid. Transfer to a colander to allow excess liquid to drain, 4 to 5 minutes. Transfer to a large bowl and toss with the sauce. Garnish with the seaweed and serve immediately.

2½ pounds zucchini or yellow squash, or a combination of squash and beets

6 scallions, thinly sliced

Zest and juice of 1 orange

½ cup low-sodium tamari

¼ cup honey or agave nectar, or 2 tablespoons stevia

1 tablespoon cider vinegar

2 tablespoons sesame oil

2 garlic cloves, minced

1 teaspoon minced fresh ginger

2 teaspoons cornstarch

1 teaspoon chili garlic sauce

1 teaspoon freshly ground black pepper

Olive oil cooking spray

2 (0.5-ounce) packages seaweed chips, thinly sliced

per serving
207 calories
5 g (1 g) fat (sat)
39 g carbs
30 g sugar
5 g fiber
8 g protein
767 mg sodium

Brazil nuts are the "it" food if you want to replenish your selenium, a supernutrient for the thyroid. But limit yourself to four nuts per day. Baking them in a spicy butter adds soulful flavors and complements the inherent tang of the nuts.

BUTTERED
Brazil Nuts

SERVES 16

Cooking spray

¼ cup coconut sugar

1 tablespoon unsalted grass-fed butter or coconut or olive oil

¼ teaspoon garlic salt

¼ teaspoon dried chipotle chile

¼ teaspoon freshly ground black pepper

2 cups whole Brazil nuts

Coat a baking sheet or toaster oven tray with cooking spray. Preheat an oven or toaster oven to 350°F. Place the coconut sugar, butter, and ¼ cup of warm water in large skillet over medium heat. Cook, stirring once or twice, for 1 to 2 minutes, or until the mixture thickens. Add the garlic salt, chipotle chile, black pepper, and nuts, tossing well. Remove from the heat and transfer to a tray to cool completely before serving or transfer to an airtight container and store, refrigerated, up to 1 month.

4 Brazil nuts
121 *calories*
12 g (3 g) *fat (sat)*
4 g *carbs*
2 g *sugar*
1 g *fiber*
2 g *protein*
31 mg *sodium*

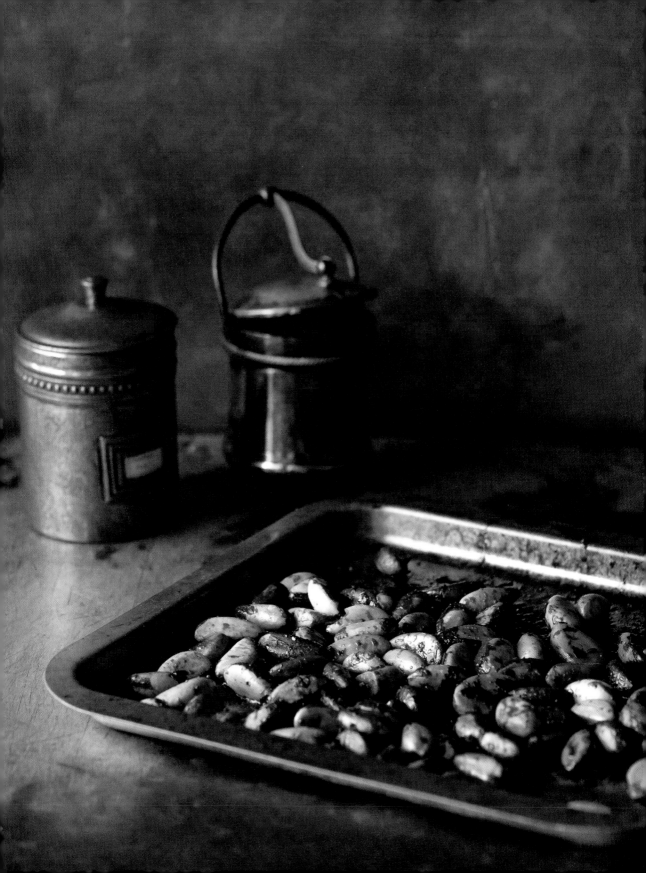

Essential Oil Preparations and Rituals for Fermentation

DIFFUSER OIL BLEND FOR SELF-EXPRESSION

This chapter focuses on healing for the throat and having clear nasal passages is part of expressing yourself clearly. Try this essential oil blend in your diffuser, before a big presentation or a difficult heart-to-heart talk with a loved one. This blend is also great to diffuse while you practice the "decree" meditations on page 171.

3 drops tea tree essential oil

3 drops eucalyptus essential oil

Fill your essential oil diffuser with water according to the diffuser instructions. Add the oils and turn on the mister.

DIFFUSER OIL BLEND FOR SWEET TALK

Part of "speaking your truth" and "speaking your mind" is to do it with finesse and kindness. Meditate on this idea as you enjoy this unusual oil blend, where a hint of sweet jasmine softens astringent tea tree oil.

4 drops tea tree essential oil

1 drop jasmine essential oil

Fill your essential oil diffuser with water according to the diffuser instructions. Add the oils and turn on the mister.

MINTY COCONUT OIL TOOTHPASTE

Keeping your breath fresh is one way to feel more confident about speaking, whether you are speaking to someone you've long admired or giving your first public speech. Mint oil disinfects and gives you that minty scent you expect from toothpaste.

MAKES ⅓ CUP TOOTHPASTE

¼ cup coconut oil

3 tablespoons baking soda

1 teaspoon stevia

4 drops mint oil

2 drops orange, lemon, or chamomile essential oil

Place the coconut oil, baking soda, stevia, mint oil, and orange oil in a small bowl. Mix with a rubber spatula until smooth. Use as you would toothpaste. Store in an airtight container, refrigerated, for up to 2 weeks.

CHAMOMILE ORANGE LIP BALM

Chapped lips are a nuisance when you're trying to express yourself, whether it's a simple chat with a friend or while doing a company-wide presentation. Depending on the texture you prefer, use 3 tablespoons of coconut oil for a more ChapStick-like texture or 4 to 5 tablespoons for a creamier balm.

MAKES 10 LIP BALMS

10 (10 ml) lip balm containers

¼ cup (2 ounces) white beeswax pellets

3 to 4 tablespoons unrefined coconut oil

1 tablespoon jojoba oil

5 drops chamomile essential oil

5 drops pure wild orange essential oil

1 teaspoon pure vanilla extract

Remove the lids from the lip balm containers and line up the empty containers on the counter.

Place the beeswax pellets in the top of a double boiler over medium-low heat. Once the water starts to boil, reduce the heat to low and stir the beeswax constantly until it is completely melted with no lumps, 5 to 6 minutes. The melting time will vary depending on which type of beeswax you are using.

Stir in the coconut oil, jojoba oil, chamomile and orange essential oils, and vanilla. Stir until the oils are well incorporated and the mixture is smooth.

Leave the double boiler on the lowest heat to keep the mixture warm while you fill your lip balm containers, using a teaspoon, since the beeswax mixture can harden quickly. Allow the lip balm to set for about hour, on the countertop, then top with the lids.

NOTES: When you first add the vanilla, it will dot the solution, but don't be concerned as it will incorporate as the beeswax dissolves.

To clean up spills easily, Bar Keepers Friend is a gentle cleanser that will remove the beeswax without scratching surfaces.

If using a Pyrex container when pouring the wax, fill it with hot water and use a cloth to wipe it clean. It's best to have a dedicated container for wax making.

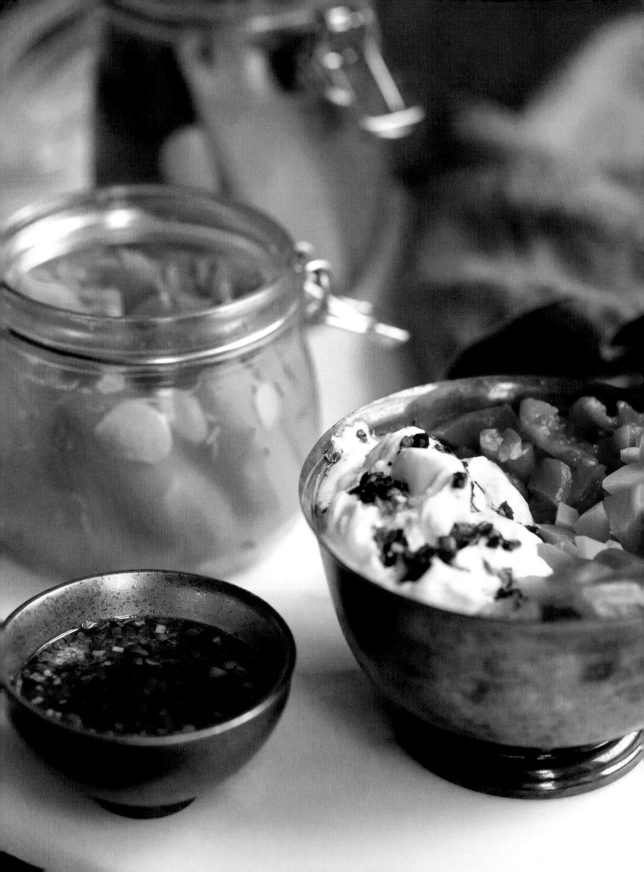

Decree Meditation to Activate the Voice

The health of your thyroid greatly effects the quality and sound of your voice. Beyond protecting your physical voice, your voice can be used on a psychological level as a tool for emotional well-being and a way to feel more connected to others. Feeling good about using your voice and hearing the sound of your own voice can bring about a healthier emotional state. Proper diaphragmatic breathing, important in mediation, is key to having the most attractive-sounding, commanding voice that can draw others to you.

Decreeing, or declaring your wishes out loud, is an energy-boosting way to kick-start manifesting goals, since voicing your emotions creates a feedback loop that can help you see things more objectively. It can be considered a more advanced spiritual practice, since many people fear saying things aloud, due to a wide range of mental or emotional blocks. In many cases, these blocks are created by childhood experiences that internalized the ideas that "speaking up is bad" or "I don't have a right to voice my thoughts." When you first learn to decree, it can feel a bit embarrassing or strange at first, especially if you are shy or reserved, but voicing your intent, like writing, has real psychological benefits: hearing your intention aloud helps seed or reinforce the subconscious mind with the idea, setting you up to feel more positive about taking the action needed to achieve your goals.

This meditation practice will help you to become more accustomed to speaking your thoughts and feelings aloud. Choose a mantra or saying of your choice, it should be something positive and very specific to what you wish to manifest.

Healing Stone Therapy
Aquamarine, azurite, and lapis lazuli are all healing crystals for this area. While practicing any of the meditations featured in this book you can rest one of these crystals in the divot between the collarbones called the suprasternal notch. Most jewelers will set any of these stones to make a choker-length necklace, ideal for activating the throat energy center.

If you are shy or feel awkward speaking your mantra aloud, plan this exercise in a private room or at home when you're alone. Find a comfortable seat, cross-legged on the floor or seated in a chair with your legs uncrossed and feet firmly planted on the floor. Close your eyes and begin to breathe deeply through your nose. Feel your belly rise and fall initiating the breath from your stomach. Continue to breathe from the stomach, expanding it first, and then slowing down the breath to a count of four while you clear you mind and relax the body. Gently open your eyes and say your decree aloud, whichever sentence or mantra you selected. You can whisper it at first to "break the seal" of past conditioning, but continue to repeat it as you get louder and louder. You may feel heat rising in the body, and this is a normal physiological reaction, as you increase the volume of your voice. After you have spoken the decree at least seven times, relax and return to normal breathing.

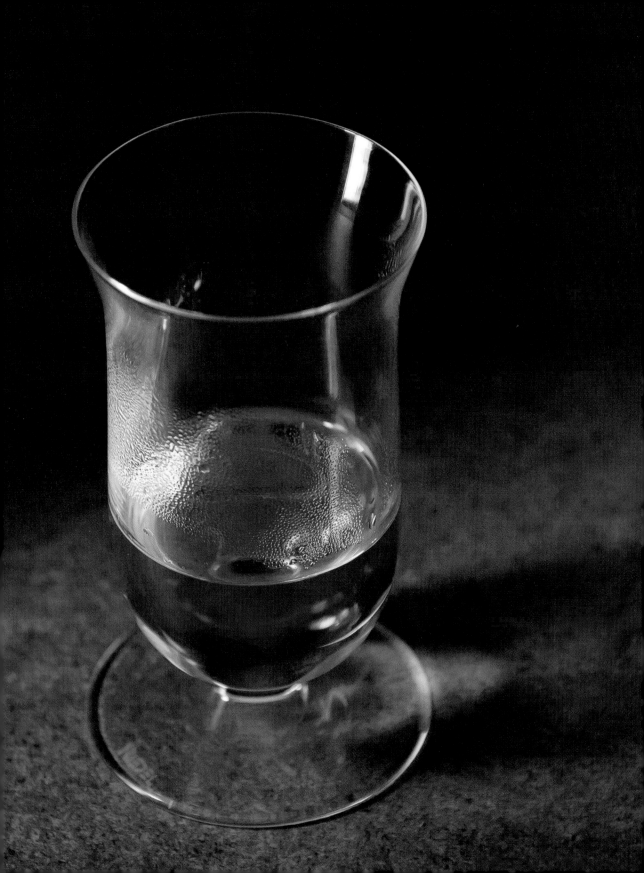

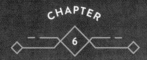

CHAPTER 6

Distillation

FOCUSING AND CALMING THE MIND

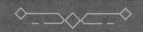

Do you feel like your brain is in a constant fog? "Brain fog," a fairly new health term, is a type of mental fatigue that can show up as lack of focus, poor memory, and feelings of confusion. Most people credit brain fog to stress and being overworked, but it may also be the result of a malnourished brain, according to integrated psychiatrists. The foods in this chapter contain brain-boosting nutrients that can help. I also recommend daily mindful meditations and "brain breaks," such as the essential oil therapies on page 200.

You may be familiar with the term distillation as part of the purification process for alcoholic beverages, but the word can also be used in a mental/emotional sense. In alchemy, this is a stage where refining takes place, and where you become clear on large goals, life purpose, and plans. So, alongside foods to help dispel brain fog, the rituals and meditation for this chapter will help you to gain more clarity and overcome unhealthful habits. Apart from working more efficiently, by gaining more clarity you can get a handle on the "bigger picture," or what you really want for your life along with the steps necessary to achieve life goals.

For the ancient Egyptians (who created alchemy), the two major brain glands, pituitary and pineal, were considered the most sacred. They saw them as the seat of power to the health of the body and a way to connect to divine energies linked to thoughts and feelings. This chapter focuses on the pituatary; the pituitary rules over your endocrine system, which includes all the glands and hormones they make to operate your entire body. The pituitary gland is housed in the hypothalamus, a communication region that also has the important job of controlling memory, emotional balance, body temperature, food intake, water intake, and how well you sleep.

Proper care for this energy center involves a combination of eating properly, having proper sleep hygiene (since that's when it secretes human growth hormone, HGH—see also Chapter 7, Solidification), and meditation while limiting foods that harm your cognitive powers and your brain, including processed sugar, white carbohydrates, harmful fats, and too much alcohol. The recipes in this chapter are made with healthier fats—the kinds you'll find in olive oil, dark chocolate, and walnuts. The cooking fats that you'll find in this chapter and throughout the book have unique molecular structures that can boost overall healing and help cognition—and they are flavorful, to boot! What makes them healing is their fatty acid profile, which has been widely researched. These recipes include fats, such as coconut oil (boasting medium-chain triglycerides [MCTs]), grass-fed dairy (which is surprisingly high in omega-3s), and olive and sesame oils (both of which contain high amounts of both mono- and polyunsaturated fats). Enjoying these oils in moderate amounts makes the perfect synergistic pairing for nutrient-dense superfoods, medicinal foods, and adaptogens. These types of fats also have a mild antioxidant effect in the body, and are a delicious way to help increase bioabsorption of fat-soluble vitamins A and D, among others, as well as uptake of some of the power molecules found in medicinal and adaptogenic plants (such as the curcumin molecules in turmeric).

Superfoods, Herbs, and Essential Oils for the Brain and Pituitary Gland

BLUEBERRIES: Many studies have linked blueberries to brain health due to their polyphenols, in particular anthocyanin. Anthocyanin is especially good for your brain since it can pass through the blood-brain barrier and help neurons communicate more efficiently.

WALNUTS: One of the oldest tree foods known to man, the King of Nuts outranks all other nuts, except pecans, in antioxidants, which are found in their skins. Walnuts also contain high amounts of polyunsaturated fats that help maintain neuronal membrane integrity.

COFFEE: Coffee is made from the bean of a tropical shrub that grows close to the ground. It ranks high in antioxidants and is being studied in connection to cognitive function. Most of the benefits come from a synergy of the neuroprotective qualities in caffeine paired with antioxidants that zap free radicals.

DARK CHOCOLATE: Dark chocolate containing at least 70% ground cacao beans boasts healing flavonols that cross the blood-brain barrier and help ensure the survival of neurons. These flavonols are also known to increase blood flow in the part of the brain that controls memory. Dark chocolate is also a good source of plant-based iron, essential for blood flow and necessary for the growth of your brain's white matter.

NUTMEG AND NUTMEG OIL: Nutmeg has been studied for its potential to boost cognition and protect the tissues of the brain. Nutmeg contains myristicin and elemicin, which together can soothe and gently stimulate areas of your brain.

ROSEMARY AND ROSEMARY ESSENTIAL OIL: A fragrant herb with evergreenlike leaves, rosemary is part of the mint family. The herb and its essential oil have been used for memory in folk medicine and herbalism, and a few small studies confirm these results. It contains carnosic acid, which has been shown to be very detoxifying for the brain.

SAGE AND CLARY SAGE OIL: Like rosemary, sage is considered to be a memory enhancer. Compounds in sage may protect the brain against degenerative diseases. Sage contains a "cocktail" of neural protective compounds called polyphenolic acids that are antioxidant, antidepressant, anti-inflammatory, and neurotropic.

SANDALWOOD ESSENTIAL OIL: Bearing a woodsy yet sweet fragrance, sandalwood has been used for centuries in Eastern religious ceremonies. Like most essential oils, sandalwood has antibacterial and antifungal properties.

Chai, which simply means "tea" in Hindi, is used traditionally to awaken for the day's duties and sharpen the mind. Using coffee in place of tea with this traditional spiced drink gives it a richer, more complex taste and even more power to banish brain fog. The key to enjoying coffee the healthy way is to drink it in moderation—three cups or less a day—and if you have any health conditions, check with your doctor to see whether caffeine is safe for you.

BANISH BRAIN FOG
Chai Coffee

SERVES 2

4 tablespoons ground dark roast coffee beans

½ teaspoon ground green cardamom

½ teaspoon ground cinnamon

¼ teaspoon freshly grated nutmeg

1 cup grass-fed whole milk or coconut milk

Place the coffee in a coffeemaker along with the cardamom, cinnamon, and nutmeg and brew according to the manufacturer's instructions. Gently warm the milk in a small saucepan over low heat. Stir the warm milk into the coffee and serve.

per serving
44 *calories*
3 g (2 g) *fat (sat)*
4 g *carbs*
3 g *sugar*
0 g *fiber*
0 g *protein*
23 mg *sodium*

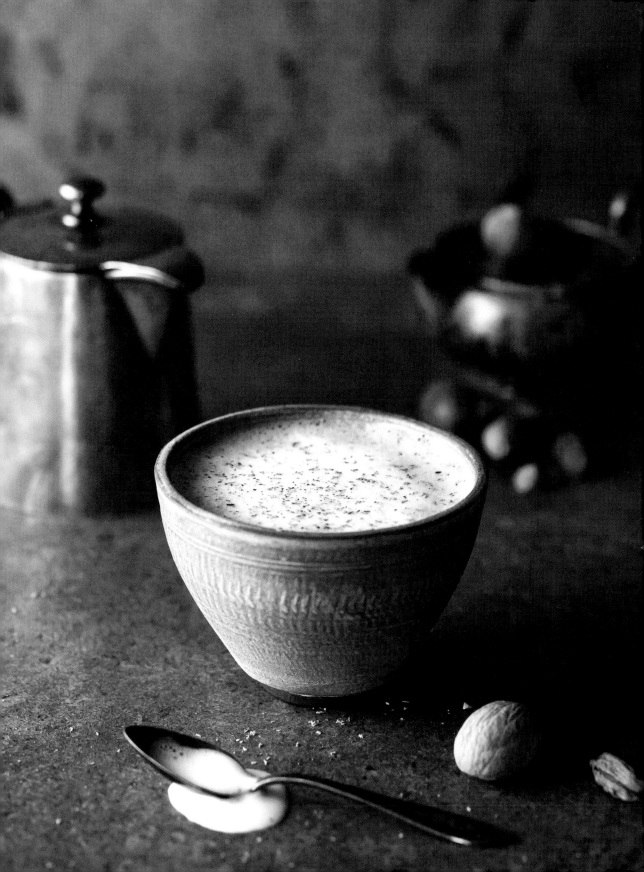

Hemp is a great way to get all eight of your essential amino acids in one fell swoop or, in this case, one tasty glass! Blueberries have the compound anthocyanin, which has many health benefits—it is found in high quantities in blue, red, and purple superfoods featured throughout this book. Combining hemp and berries makes this sweet smoothie a nutritional powerhouse—and a beautiful creamy blue.

BLUEBERRY HEMP
Cardamom Smoothie

SERVES 2

2 cup fresh or frozen blueberries

2 cups baby spinach

⅔ cup protein powder or Greek yogurt

1 cup grass-fed dairy milk or coconut milk

2 tablespoons hemp seeds

½ teaspoons ground cardamom

8 ice cubes

Place the blueberries, spinach, protein powder, milk, hemp seeds, cardamom, and ice in a blender and process until smooth. Divide between two glasses and serve immediately.

per serving
321 *calories*
11 g (4 g) *fat (sat)*
36 g *carbs*
22 g *sugar*
9 g *fiber*
26 g *protein*
172 mg *sodium*

Tired of drinking that same old cup of coffee in the morning? Try this smoothie, which is like breakfast in a glass. Cacao has been shown to have positive benefits on the arteries in your brain and heart. If you don't have the chilled coffee on hand, you can use 1 tablespoon of instant coffee. If you aren't a regular coffee drinker, or you're looking to try something different, you can try mushroom-infused instant coffee, instead: these potent beverage blends, made from different medicinal mushrooms, support your energy and stamina and give a good dose of antioxidants without all the caffeine.

Mocha Chip Smoothie
WITH CACAO NIBS

Place the protein powder, banana, milk, coffee, nuts, ice cubes, and cacao nibs in a blender and process until smooth. Divide between two glasses and serve immediately.

SERVES 2

⅔ cup protein powder or plain Greek or coconut yogurt

1 banana

½ cup grass-fed dairy milk or coconut milk

½ cup strongly brewed coffee, chilled

2 tablespoons walnuts or macadamia nuts

8 ice cubes

2 tablespoons cacao nibs, or 2 squares dark 70% cacao chocolate

per serving
359 *calories*
26 g (17 g) *fat (sat)*
24 g *carbs*
13 g *sugar*
5 g *fiber*
12 g *protein*
44 mg *sodium*

Want a fun way to eat cauliflower? Slice it into thick pieces and serve it like steak. The drizzle of balsamic reduction or *saba* (an Italian syrup made from wine must) adds sweet acidity while a sprinkle of cacao nibs fortifies the dish with antioxidants. You can buy saba, also known as *vin cotto* or *mosto cotto*, on the Internet, as it may not be available at your local grocery store.

Charred Cauliflower
WITH CACAO NIBS AND ROSEMARY

SERVES 4

½ cup balsamic vinegar, or 4 tablespoons store-bought balsamic crema or saba

2 large heads cauliflower (about 5 pounds)

4 tablespoons olive or coconut oil

½ teaspoon salt

¼ cup cacao nibs

2 teaspoons finely minced rosemary leaves

2 teaspoons unsweetened cocoa powder

In a well-ventilated kitchen, prepare a balsamic reduction (skip this step if using store-bought balsamic crema or saba): Place the vinegar in a small saucepan over medium-low heat and simmer for 15 to 20 minutes, or until it thickens to the consistency of maple syrup. Remove from the heat and set aside while you prepare the cauliflower. The mixture will continue to thicken as it cools.

Remove the any leaves around the cauliflower heads and trim the stem ends, but keep the heads intact. Place on a cutting board, stem side down, and cut both heads into thick steak-size slabs about 1½ inches thick. Place two skillets (be sure you have a lid for each pan, though you are not using those yet) over medium heat and heat 2 tablespoons of the oil in each skillet. Divide the cauliflower slices between the two skillets. Sprinkle ¼ teaspoon of the salt into each skillet.

Cook the cauliflower for 10 to 15 minutes, turning occasionally, or until it starts to char. Reduce the heat to low, cover, and cook for an additional 10 to 15 minutes, or until fork-tender. Drizzle with the balsamic reduction, balsamic crema, or saba. Sprinkle with the cacao nibs, rosemary, and cocoa powder. Serve immediately.

— ◇ —
per serving
360 calories
21 g (6 g) *fat (sat)*
37 g carbs
16 g sugar
13 g fiber
12 g protein
468 mg sodium
— ◇ —

THE SUPERFOOD ALCHEMY COOKBOOK

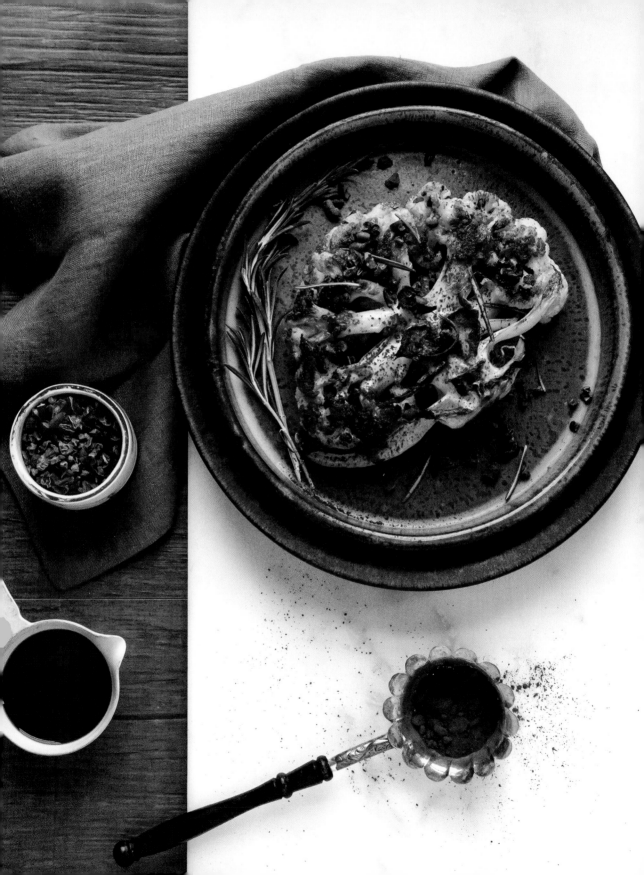

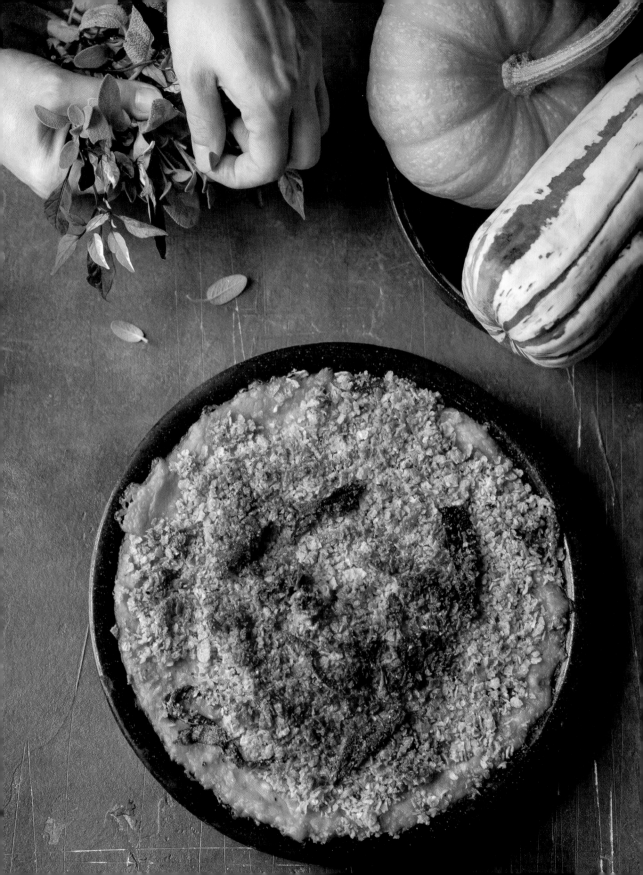

The creamy texture of cooked butternut squash is combined with the rich, sweet flavor of coconut milk to create a dish packed with warming fall flavors. In addition to being a brain superspice, nutmeg helps improve liver and kidney function and may be used to prevent and dissolve kidney stones. This dish pairs perfectly with a hot cup of herbal tea or mulled spiced wine for entertaining.

SIMPLE
Squash Sage Gratin

Place the butternut squash puree, milk, nutmeg, salt, and pepper in a large bowl and stir until well combined. Spoon into an 8 by 8-inch baking dish or 9-inch pie plate.

Place the butter in a large skillet over medium heat. Add the herbs and cook for 3 to 4 minutes, or until they start to crisp. Toss in the cornflakes and cook for 1 to 2 minutes more, stirring well to toast them.

Sprinkle the cornflake mixture over the top of the squash. Sprinkle the Parmesan over the cornflakes, then transfer to the oven. Bake for 25 to 30 minutes, or until the top is golden brown and the squash is hot. Serve immediately.

1 (15-ounce) can butternut squash puree

1 cup coconut milk, or ½ cup heavy cream

½ teaspoon freshly grated nutmeg

¼ teaspoon salt

¼ teaspoon freshly ground black pepper

1 tablespoon unsalted grass-fed butter or olive oil

¼ cup packed fresh sage

¼ cup packed fresh rosemary leaves

1 cup crushed cornflakes or gluten-free bread crumbs

½ cup grated Parmesan cheese (optional)

---

per serving
268 calories
17 g (11 g) fat (sat)
25 g carbs
1 g sugar
1 g fiber
7 g protein
413 mg sodium

Traditional mole is notorious among home and pro cooks alike for its complicated preparation. This recipe keeps the complex flavors of this Mexican dream sauce but ditches the complex cookery. Chocolate is known to have many health benefits, one of which is that it contains flavanols, which may help lower blood pressure.

Shortcut Chocolate Mole
WITH ROOT VEGETABLES

SERVES 4

2 sweet potatoes, peeled and diced

1 pound carrots, peeled and cut into spears

1 pound parsnips, peeled and cut into spears

½ cup vegetable stock

½ cup cashew or peanut butter

½ cup raisins

¼ cup sesame seeds

2 tablespoons chipotle chile in adobo

4 garlic cloves, cut in half

Juice of 2 oranges

2 tablespoons cider vinegar

1 teaspoon salt

2 ounces dark 70% chocolate

Place the sweet potatoes, carrots, and parsnips in the slow cooker set to HIGH while you prepare the rest of the recipe.

Place the stock, nut butter, raisins, sesame seeds, chipotle chile, garlic, orange juice, vinegar, and salt in a blender or food processor and process until smooth. Transfer to the slow cooker and change the setting to LOW. Cook for 2 to 2½ hours, or until the sauce thickens and the sweet potatoes are tender.

During the last 10 minutes of cooking, add the chocolate and cover, to allow to melt. Stir once or twice before serving.

per serving
574 *calories*
27 g (7 g) *fat (sat)*
78 g *carbs*
37 g *sugar*
15 g *fiber*
13 g *protein*
914 mg *sodium*

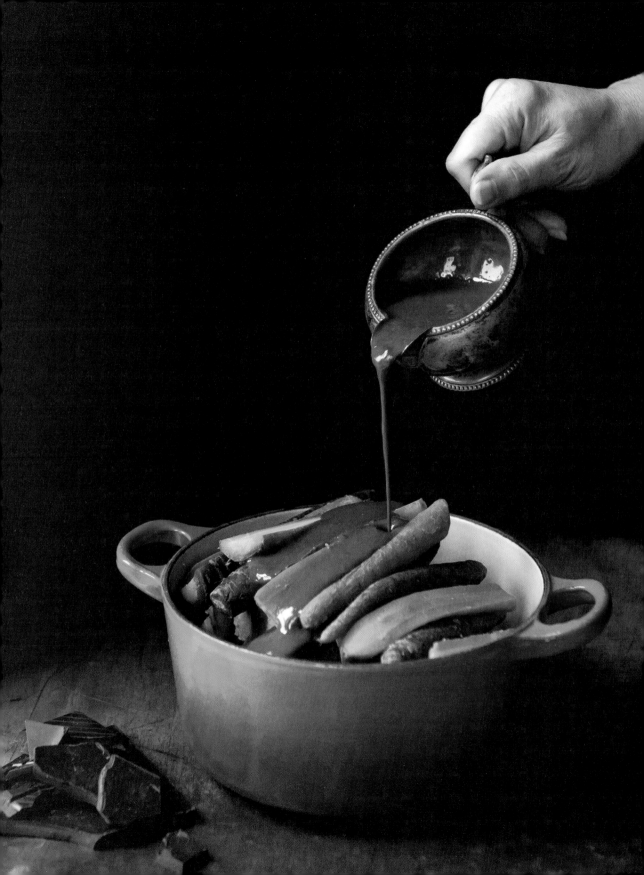

Nothing could be more satisfying than a crispy, herb-enhanced handful of nuts on top of a warm, creamy root vegetable soup. Cauliflower is among the creamiest, and full of sulforaphanes that help protect the body against disease and inflammation. Serve this piping hot out of the pot and you'll be sure to warm the heart of whoever gets the bowl.

Cream of Cauliflower Soup
WITH ROSEMARY-CRUSTED PECANS

SERVES 4

2 tablespoons plus 1 teaspoon unsalted grass-fed butter or olive oil

1 onion, diced

4 celery stalks, diced

2 carrots, diced

2 tablespoons gluten-free multipurpose flour

1 head cauliflower, cut into florets

5 cups vegetable stock

½ cup pecans

1 tablespoon chopped fresh rosemary leaves

¼ cup heavy cream or coconut cream

¼ cup thinly sliced chives or scallions

Heat the 2 tablespoons of the butter in a large stockpot over medium heat. Add the onion, celery, and carrots. Cook, stirring often, for 8 to 10 minutes, or until the vegetables are tender. Add the cauliflower and stock. Bring to a simmer over medium heat, cover, and cook for 12 to 15 minutes, or until the cauliflower is tender.

While the soup is cooking, prepare the pecans: Heat the remaining teaspoon of butter in a small skillet over medium heat and add the pecans and rosemary. Cook, stirring often, for 2 to 3 minutes, or until the pecans start to become fragrant.

Remove from the heat.

When the cauliflower is tender, remove the soup from heat and let cool for 5 minutes, then add the cream.

Blend the soup with an immersion blender, or carefully blend in batches in a standing blender or food processor, until smooth. Divide the soup among four bowls. Top with the chives and pecans and serve immediately.

1¾ cups	
226	calories
14 g (9 g)	fat (sat)
17 g	carbs
5 g	sugar
4 g	fiber
10 g	protein
567 mg	sodium

Carrot, apple, and nutmeg are perhaps the most perfect trio for providing comfort and nourishment through the cooler seasons. Carrot famously contains beta-carotene, which the body converts into vitamin A, also known as retinol, to improve immunity and eye and skin health. Nutmeg is a stimulating brain tonic, and also helpful for detoxification and pain relief.

Roasted Carrot Apple Soup
WITH NUTMEG

SERVES 4

Heat the oil in a large stockpot over medium heat. Add the onion, garlic, black pepper, and cayenne (if using) and cook for 3 to 5 minutes. Add the carrots and apple, stirring to coat with the oil. Add the stock, lower the heat to a simmer, and cover. Simmer for 40 to 45 minutes, or until carrots are tender. Remove from the heat and stir in ½ teaspoon of the nutmeg. Let cool slightly.

Blend the soup with an immersion blender, or carefully blend in batches in a standing blender or food processor, until smooth. If soup is too thick, add ¼ to ½ cup of water to reach your desired thickness. Divide among 4 bowls and top each with a tablespoon of the sour cream and ½ teaspoon of the remaining nutmeg.

3 tablespoons olive oil or unsalted grass-fed butter

1 small onion, finely chopped

2 garlic cloves, thinly sliced

¼ to ½ teaspoon freshly ground black pepper

¼ teaspoon cayenne pepper (optional)

1 pound carrots, peeled and chopped (about 8)

1 apple, cored and diced

1 quart vegetable stock

2½ teaspoons freshly grated nutmeg

4 tablespoons sour cream or coconut creamer

per serving
282 *calories*
16 g (4 g) *fat (sat)*
29 g *carbs*
15 g *sugar*
5 g *fiber*
8 g *protein*
433 mg *sodium*

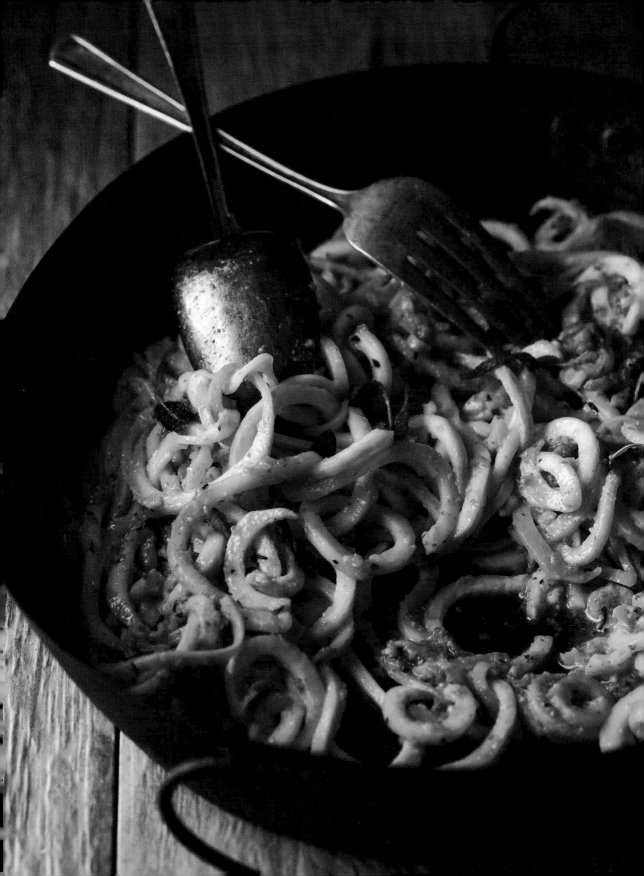

Pesto is a classic Italian sauce and a great way to utilize any fresh herbs you have lying around from other recipes. Just toss them in a food processor to create your own delicious spin on the dish. Sage contains antioxidant compounds that make it great at reducing inflammation, and it tastes great crisped by the skillet.

Walnut Pesto
OVER SQUASH NOODLES AND FRIED SAGE

Place the walnuts, lemon thyme, rosemary, lemon zest, garlic, salt, and pepper in a food processor. Pulse ten to fifteen times, or until the walnuts are finely chopped. Add the ¼ cup olive oil and pulse for 2 to 3 minutes more, or until a thick sauce forms. Stir in the Parmesan.

Using a vegetables noodle maker, process the squash into noodles. Coat a large skillet with cooking spray and heat over medium-high heat. Add the vegetable noodles and cook, tossing often, for 2 to 3 minutes, or until the noodles are tender. Transfer to a colander to drain for 4 to 5 minutes. Toss with the pesto. In the same skillet used for the noodles add remaining 1 tablespoon olive oil. Heat over medium-high heat, then add the sage leaves and cook, turning once or twice, for 2 to 3 minutes, or until the leaves are crisp. Place on top of the noodles and serve immediately.

SERVES 4

½ cup walnuts, toasted

2 tablespoons fresh
lemon thyme leaves

1 tablespoon fresh rosemary

Zest of 1 lemon

1 garlic clove, peeled
and quartered

½ teaspoon salt

¼ teaspoon freshly ground
black pepper

¼ cup plus 1 tablespoon olive oil

¼ cup grated Parmesan cheese,
or 2 tablespoons nutritional
yeast

4 yellow squash or zucchini

Cooking spray

1 cup fresh sage leaves

---◇---

per serving
377 *calories*
31 g (4 g) *fat (sat)*
20 g *carbs*
6 g *sugar*
5 g *fiber*
11 g *protein*
387 mg *sodium*

---◇---

189

Nuts are a great source of vitamins and nutrients and are just plain tasty snacks. This recipe amps up the flavor with coffee, which is one of the most easily accessed sources of antioxidants we have. Roasting the nuts helps deepen their natural flavor, adding complexity. My favorite nut mixture for this recipe includes pecans, because their texture improves to an airy crunch upon roasting. Experiment with your favorite nuts and enjoy!

Coffee-Glazed Nuts

SERVES 6

Cooking spray

½ cup strongly brewed coffee

3 tablespoons coconut sugar

2 tablespoons honey or agave nectar

2 cups whole mixed nuts

1 tablespoon finely chopped fresh rosemary

2 tablespoons unsalted grass-fed butter or coconut oil

¼ teaspoon kosher salt

Preheat the oven to 350°F. Coat a baking sheet with cooking spray. Place the coffee, sugar, and honey in a small saucepan along with ⅓ cup of water. Bring to a boil and cook for 4 to 5 minutes, or until the mixture reduces by half. Turn off the heat and stir in the nuts, rosemary, butter, and salt. Toss well.

Spread out the nut mixture on the prepared baking sheet. Bake for 10 to 15 minutes, or until the nuts begin to brown. Remove from the oven and let cool completely on the baking sheet, then transfer to an airtight container.

per serving
312 *calories*
24 g (3 g) *fat (sat)*
22 g *carbs*
12 g *sugar*
4 g *fiber*
8 g *protein*
107 mg *sodium*

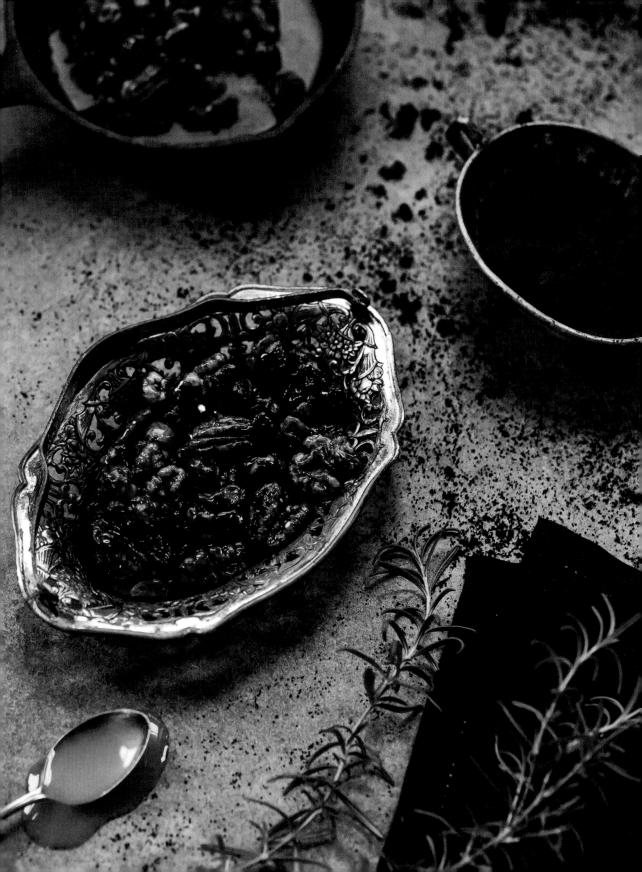

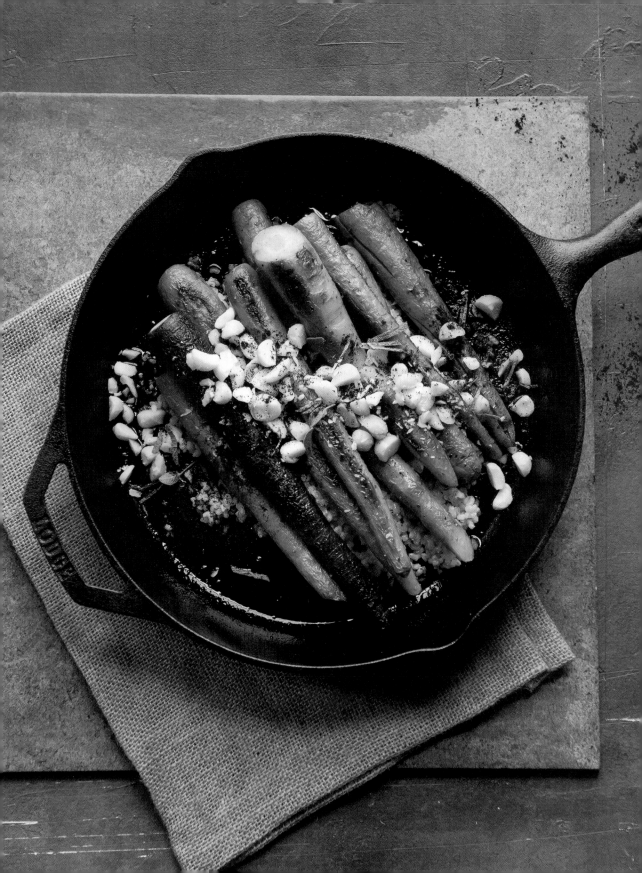

Don't toss your cold morning brew—save it, refrigerated, for this deliciously unusual recipe. Roasting carrots in the oven brings out their natural sweetness, which contrasts beautifully with bitter black coffee. The macadamia nuts give this dish not only a hint of white, like the cream in coffee, but plenty of brain-boosting monounsaturated fats.

Roasted Honey Coffee Carrots
WITH TOASTED MACADAMIA NUTS

SERVES 4

Cook the rice or quinoa according to the package instructions with the vegetable stock and set aside.

Fill a large stockpot with 3 inches of water. Cover and bring to a boil. Add the carrots and cook for 15 to 20 minutes, or until tender. Place the olive oil in a large skillet, preferably cast iron, and add the carrots. Sprinkle with the salt and cook over medium-high heat for 4 to 5 minutes, or until the carrots are golden. Transfer to a plate. Place the skillet back over low heat. Add the coffee, honey, and vinegar, cooking until a thick sauce forms. Spoon the rice or quinoa into the skillet and top with the carrots. Sprinkle with the macadamia nuts and serve immediately.

1 cup uncooked short-grain brown rice or quinoa

2 cups vegetable stock

1 pound carrots, peeled

2 tablespoons olive oil

½ teaspoon salt

½ cup strongly brewed coffee

¼ cup honey or agave nectar

1 tablespoon cider vinegar

¼ cup macadamia nuts, chopped

per serving
290 calories
14 g (2 g) *fat (sat)*
41 g *carbs*
24 g *sugar*
5 g *fiber*
3 g *protein*
801 mg *sodium*

193

Potato gnocchi can be tricky to make, but by using sweet potatoes instead the dough is more forgiving and contains far more nutrients, including vitamins A and B$_6$. Fried herbs provide plenty of flavor along with extra antioxidants and a hint of added crunch.

NUTMEG
Sweet Potato Gnocchi
WITH FRIED SAGE AND BROWN BUTTER

**SERVES 6; ABOUT
8 GNOCCHI EACH**

2 sweet potatoes, peeled and cubed

1 cup gluten-free multipurpose flour

1 tablespoon tapioca starch or cornstarch

1 teaspoon baking soda

½ teaspoon salt

½ teaspoon freshly grated nutmeg

3 tablespoons unsalted grass-fed butter or coconut oil

1 cup sage leaves

1 tablespoon fresh oregano leaves

Place the cubed sweet potatoes in a medium-size saucepan and cover with water. Bring to a boil over high heat, then lower the heat to a simmer and cover. Cook for 20 to 25 minutes, or until the sweet potatoes are fork-tender. Drain and mash with fork or handheld masher, then let cool for 4 minutes. Meanwhile, place the flour, tapioca, baking soda, salt, and nutmeg in a large bowl and stir well. Add the mashed sweet potato.

Using a large spoon or your hands, fold the ingredients together to form a sticky dough. Roll the dough into a thick, even rope and chop sharply with a paring knife into 1-inch pieces. Bring a large stockpot of water to a boil. Using a tea-spoon, drop pieces of the dough into the water and cook for 2 to 3 minutes, or until the dough floats to the top of the pot. (You may need to do this in batches to avoid overcrowding the pot.) Transfer with a slotted spoon to a shallow bowl. Repeat until all the gnocchi are cooked.

Heat the butter in a large skillet over medium heat. Add the sage and oregano and cook for 3 to 4 minutes, or until the herbs start to crisp. Add the gnocchi and toss well to coat, cooking for 2 to 3 minutes more. Serve immediately.

per serving
228 *calories*
9 g (6 g) *fat (sat)*
33 g *carbs*
3 g *sugar*
1 g *fiber*
4 g *protein*
439 mg *sodium*

194

Chocolate has a long history as a medicinal and ceremonial food for the ancient Mesoamerican people, including the Maya, Olmec, and Aztecs. Once it was exported to Spain in the sixteenth century, it quickly gained notoriety as a medicinal food and was in fact prescribed widely by Spanish physicians to treat a variety of issues, including fatigue, liver disorders, and low libido. Although modern candy bars are a far cry from the therapeutic preparations of the past, chocolate made from at least 70% cacao beans is still considered a superfood and offers memory-boosting compounds. This easy-to-make chocolate bark contains the goodness of many healing foods. The nuts and seeds are rich in magnesium and manganese that can banish brain fog, since they increase blood flow and balance blood pressure. The flowers not only add antioxidants from the pigments found in their petals, but they also provide a pleasant crunch reminiscent of a crispy candy bar.

Chocolate Nut Bark

Line an 8-inch square baking pan with parchment or waxed paper. Coat the parchment with a thin layer of cooking spray. Roughly chop all the nuts and scatter evenly in the prepared pan.

Fill a small saucepan with 2 inches of water. Fit a glass or metal bowl that rests snugly on top of the pot. The bowl should not touch the water, so reduce the amount of water in the saucepan, if needed. Bring to a simmer over low heat. Once the water is simmering, place the chocolate in the bowl.

Using a spatula, stir the chocolate occasionally, until it is melted and smooth. When fully melted, remove the bowl, using a kitchen towel or oven mitt, and pour the chocolate over the nuts. Use a rubber spatula to smooth the top of the mixture. Sprinkle with the cherries, seeds, and dried flowers. Refrigerate until set, 15 to 20 minutes. Transfer the bark to a cutting board and chop into ½ by 1-inch pieces.

MAKES ABOUT 10 DOZEN (½ BY 1-INCH) PIECES

Olive oil cooking spray

½ cup mixed nuts, such as whole hazelnuts, Brazil nuts, macadamias, or walnuts

¼ cup whole almonds

7 ounces dark 70% cacao chocolate, chopped (about 2 cups chopped)

2 tablespoons chopped dried cherries

2 tablespoons hemp or chia seeds or cacao nibs

2 tablespoons dried edible flowers, such as rose or hibiscus

½ by 1-inch piece
126 *calories*
9 g (3 g) *fat (sat)*
9 g *carbs*
3 g *sugar*
3 g *fiber*
2 g *protein*
3 mg *sodium*

195

This recipe is a play on the classic American apple pie, keeping all the flavor, but nixing the heaviness. Rosemary has been shown to help with digestion, so this is one dessert that will actually help you feel less bloated after eating it, rather than more. Feel free to experiment with various apple types as each has their own unique tastes.

HOT ROSEMARY
Apple Crumble

SERVES 6

TOPPING

¾ cup old-fashioned rolled oats

¾ cup gluten-free multipurpose flour

¼ cup stevia, or
½ cup coconut sugar

¼ teaspoon salt

3 tablespoons chilled unsalted grass-fed butter or coconut shortening, frozen

FILLING

1 tablespoon olive oil

4 apples, cored and thinly sliced

1 tablespoon finely grated ginger

2 tablespoons finely chopped rosemary

1 tablespoon cornstarch

2 tablespoons honey or agave nectar

1 teaspoon pure vanilla extract

Prepare the topping: Place the oats, flour, stevia, and salt in a large bowl. Toss well to combine. Chop the butter into small pieces and add it to the flour mixture. Rub the butter into the oat mixture until the butter pieces are the size of peas, or add the oat mixture to a food processor and pulse with the butter eight to ten times to reach the same consistency. Do not overmix. Place in the fridge while you make the filling.

Preheat the oven to 375°F.

Prepare the filling: Heat the olive oil in a large skillet over medium heat. Add the apples, ginger, and 1 tablespoon of the rosemary and cook for 10 to 15 minutes, or until the apples start to brown and soften. Lower the heat to low and sprinkle with the cornstarch.

Toss well. Add the honey or agave and vanilla along with ½ cup of water. Toss well until a thick sauce forms. Spoon the mixture into an 8 by 8-inch baking dish. Sprinkle the oat topping over the apples and transfer to the oven.

Bake until the apples are tender and the topping is brown and crisp, 40 to 45 minutes. Remove from the oven and let cool slightly. Spoon the warm crumble into bowls and serve. Garnish with remaining tablespoon of rosemary.

per serving	
321	calories
9 g (4 g)	fat (sat)
59 g	carbs
35 g	sugar
4 g	fiber
3 g	protein
107 mg	sodium

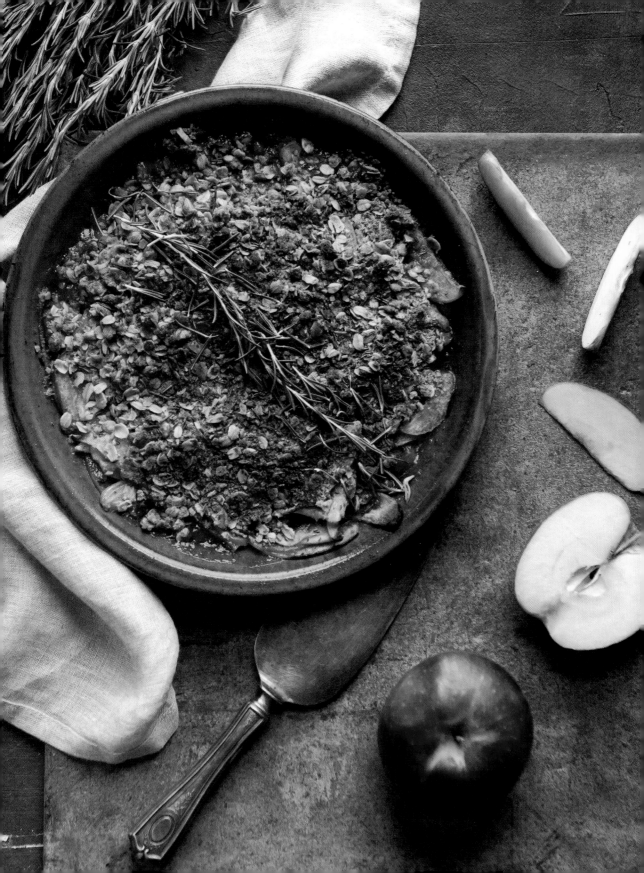

Using flavored salts in your cooking is a natural and easy way to add more flavor and enjoyment to healing foods. Consider herbs and spices to be flavor bridges between your taste buds and more nourishing superfood vegetables. Building a love relationship with healthy meals is essential to making healthy eating a more soulful, more fulfilling practice.

Flavored Herb Salts

SERVES 24

½ cup coarse salt, such as kosher

2 tablespoons chopped dried herbs, such as sage, rosemary, thyme, or dried edible flowers, such as rose, lavender, or hibiscus

Zest of 1 lemon (about 2 teaspoons) (optional)

Place the salt, herbs, and lemon zest, if using, in a small bowl. Toss well to combine and transfer to an airtight jar or container.

1 teaspoon
1 *calorie*
0 g (0 g) *fat (sat)*
0 g *carbs*
0 g *sugar*
0 g *fiber*
0 g *protein*
2,338 mg *sodium*

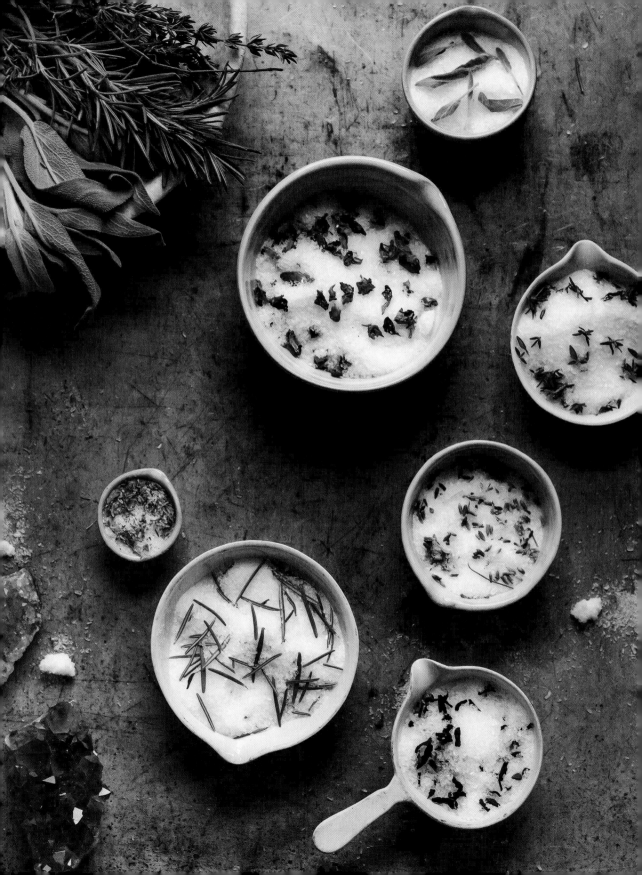

Essential Oil Preparations and Rituals for Distillation

DIFFUSER OIL BLEND TO CALM AND FOCUS

Rosemary is a super brain food that also makes an enlivening oil. Mixing it with sandalwood sweetens the blend making it more interesting.

4 drops rosemary essential oil

3 drops sandalwood essential oil

Fill your essential oil diffuser with water according to the diffuser instructions. Add the oils and turn on the mister. If you don't have lime essential oil on hand, opt for orange or lemon.

NUTMEG MASSAGE OIL

Anyone who works on a computer experiences a sore neck and shoulders and a general feeling of tightness and mental fatigue. Regular massage not only releases stress that can put a damper on clarity, but also help with boost mental health. Use this delicious massage oil to loosen up your shoulders while enrobing you in luscious scent.

1 tablespoons coconut oil

1 teaspoon sesame or jojoba oil

1 teaspoon freshly grated nutmeg, or 1 drop nutmeg essential oil

Place the coconut oil, sesame oil, and nutmeg in a small bowl and mix well with a spoon. Use immediately or store, refrigerated, for up to 2 weeks.

DIFFUSER OIL BLEND TO REFRESH THE MIND

Crave an interesting diffuser scent that can help refresh you while you meditate? Enjoy this blend that uses lime to lighten up the pinelike scent of rosemary.

4 drops rosemary essential oil

3 drops lime essential oil

Fill your essential oil diffuser with water according to the diffuser instructions. Add the oils and turn on the mister. If you don't have lime essential oil on hand, opt for orange or lemon.

THIRD EYE MEDITATION OIL

Apart from frankincense, sandalwood is considered one of the most sacred plants around, making it a great oil to use during mediation. You can also use it to scent stone mala beads or metal jewelry to provide scent to mementos you handle regularly.

1 teaspoon coconut, jojoba, or sweet almond oil

2 drops lemon essential oil

1 drop sandalwood essential oil

Place the oils in a small dish and stir to combine. Place a dot of the oil mixture between your eyebrows, also termed the "third eye" space. Enjoy any of the meditations featured in this book.

MIND-RELEASING HEAD MASSAGE

Distillation is a form of "clarifying," whether it is happening in a flask or in your mind. Head massage is a traditional Indian and Balinese therapy that will soon become your favorite after a stressful day, since it releases tension and increases blood flow, which can help you to think more clearly and improve memory. This technique does use plenty of oil directly on the head and in your hair, so plan it for a night in. You can sleep with the oil in your hair as a treatment for dry tresses; just be cautious when showering postmassage, since residual oil can make surfaces slick. You can give yourself a head massage or entreat your partner to provide one and treat him or her to one as well!

2 to 4 tablespoons coconut oil

2 to 3 drops sandalwood or sage essential oil

Place the coconut oil and sandalwood oil in small bowl and stir well with a rubber spatula or spoon until the essential oil is well combined. Drape an old towel around your shoulders. Find a comfortable seat next to a side table or another place to rest the oil. Dip your fingertips into the oil and run your fingers through your hair, scraping your scalp gently with your fingernails. Repeat until your hair is well oiled. Place your fingertips on the top of your head, allowing your thumbs to grip the base of your skull. Press your fingers into the top of your head, while dragging you thumbs up your head toward your forehead. Mix and match from the following techniques to continue massaging your head:

Make two fists. Rub the top of your head with the edges of your knuckles. Gently rub your temples with the tops of your knuckles and continue on behind your ears.

Tussle your hair by scrubbing your scalp with your fingertips.

Wisdom from Past Pains Technique

In alchemy, distillation is about seeing the big picture, resonating with higher truths and gaining more wisdom and insight, while maintaining a bit of emotional detachment. Recasting a painful situation into one that has had some benefit or potential catalyst for purpose in your life can set you free from reliving past pain that bubbles up from memories. By changing your perspective on past events, you can gain wisdom and freedom.

To begin, choose any of the essential oils from this chapter and place one drop in the palm of your right hand. Rub your hands together, creating heat and allowing the scent to blossom. Bring your hands to your nose to inhale while you take deep slow breaths in and out of the nose. Think of a past painful memory. Then think of fives way this effect has either changed your life for the better or made you a stronger, more evolved person, as you scan the body relaxing any tension that might have been trigger by negative emotions. Write down these five ways in a journal and revisit them any time you find yourself experiencing negative emotions around the specific event.

How to Dry Sage

Sage, also called salvia, has long been considered sacred. Certain compounds found in sage—carnosol and carnosic acid—can block inflammation and ease pain. Fresh sage has a strong smell and flavor (due to its protective compounds) and a small bunch goes a long way in recipes. Having leftover fresh sage can be a boon: dry it to use in cooking or use it to sage your space (see below). To dry a bundle of sage, bundle the sage stems together with a bit of twine or a rubber band. Hang it upside down in a warm room, preferably your kitchen. Allow the sage to dry until it is crumbly, about five days.

Saging Your Space

Saging or "smudging" your spaces can rid your space of harmful bacteria for up to 24 hours and creates a sense of calm while preforming this easy ritual. Whether you use your own dried sage or one you've purchased, you can perform this simple ritual any time you need to freshen up your space: after a party, after you've been ill, or even after a disagreement with a loved one or roommate, to "clean the air." To sage, start by your front door. Light

your sage bundle and blow out the flames, allowing the sage to smoke and smolder. Begin to your left, working clockwise through the room. Using your hand or a feather, "brush" the smoke in the air along the walls, lifting the bundle high and low, along the walls and into corners. Continue through the whole house, walking and saging in a clockwise fashion, relighting the bundle as needed. As you sage, set an intention to bring in fresh energy. You can do this with a simple mantra that you repeat out loud or in your head, such as "bring fresh life-giving energies" or "clear any negative energies" (create one that feels right to you as you work). Stay focused on this mantra; do not allow other thoughts to interrupt it.

Sage Tea Meditation

Sage is both stimulating and calming for the brain, enhancing memory while calming anxiety, according to a few small-scale studies. When you brew your tea for this mediation, don't use caffeinated teas, as caffeine can make the mind overactive and even cause low-grade anxiety. Sage tastes particularly good with sweeter-tasting, naturally decaffeinated teas, such as fruit teas, redbush, or hibiscus tea. Add a teaspoon of lavender honey (page 231) if you have it on hand. This practice is a great morning meditation, especially if you tend to feel rushed in the morning. Set your alarm just five minutes earlier so you can have this morning time for yourself before prepping for work.

Brew one cup of tea by steeping 1 table-spoon of fruit or any herbal, caffeine-free tea mixed with 1 tablespoon of crumbled dried sage for 4 to 5 minutes. Sit in a quiet room and allow your eyes to focus on any steam rising from the tea. Allow your eyes to close slightly as you soften your gaze. Watch the steam rising, concentrating on it to push out other thoughts, as you watch the steam form loose patterns. Continuing meditating on the steam for 2 to 3 minutes more. If you are on a schedule, set a timer so you won't feel the need to check a clock. After meditating, enjoy the tea.

Remodeling Your House Meditation

Now that you have some fundamental practices around meditation in place, you'll be on the way to building a strong mediation routine that can help support your life in a multitude of ways, like building a house with a solid foundation, room by room.

If you get "stuck" at any time or feel discourage while trying to keep up with your meditation practice, just see it as momentary stalls in construction and try to get back on track as soon as possible. Research has shown that the brain is very elastic, specifically the neurons that drive the connections and behavior in the brain. The brain can reorganize or remodel itself, so to speak, which can happen with better nutrition, new activities and exercises, and even new ways of thinking—and yes, you've guessed it—this happens with regular mediation.

What's most important with your mediation practice is not the kind of mediation

you do, but the regularity with which you practice. Just as with any sport, art, public speaking, or exercise routine, regular practice brings about amazing results. Begin with the calming breath work on page 239 before you begin this mediation.

Healing Stone Therapy

Amethyst, moonstone, and fluorite are all healing crystals for this area. While practicing any of the meditations featured in this book, you can rest one of these crystals between your brows. To add scent, simply rub your crystal with the "Third Eye Meditation Oil" or any oil from this chapter.

Now you are ready to remodel your house. Throughout this visualization, continue your slow and steady breath work. Imagine that your body is a house. Your legs, arms, torso, neck, and head are all rooms in your house. Some rooms may be clean with functioning appliances or new furniture, while others might need some work. Scan the rooms of your house to see which ones need cleansing or remodeling without judgments or emotions, simply observing. As you take in your deep breaths, start with the room that needs the most repair, and send breath to that part of your body. See that space as a room that you are cleaning. Perhaps you are tidying up or washing items in that room, setting things straight that may have fallen, or repairing broken pieces of furniture. If thoughts come into your mind, allow them to float out like passing clouds over your house. Continue to concentrate on the breath and the music. When the music ends, you can slowly open your eyes, feeling refreshed and healed.

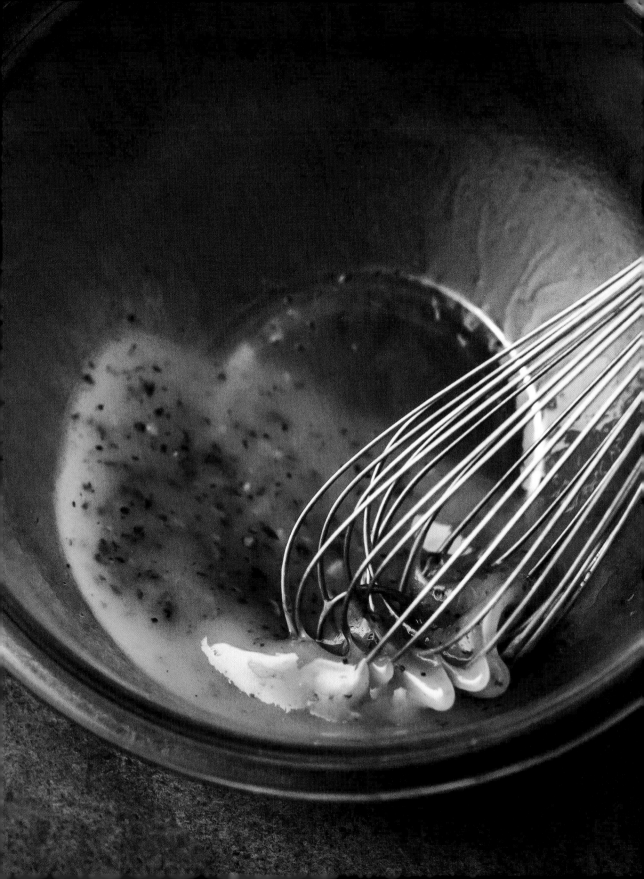

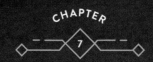
Solidification

STRENGTHENING THE NERVOUS AND IMMUNE SYSTEMS

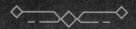

Our modern lifestyles—the long work hours, processed foods, little sleep, and overuse of alcohol and caffeine—chip away at our nervous and immune systems every day. Pollution, the "nervous" and addictive energy created by computers, hectic commutes, and the fast-paced world around us also contribute. While we can't control the stressors the world throws at us, strengthening and bringing balance to these systems is a fantastic way to alleviate the effects of stress on the body and mind.

The recipes and therapies in this chapter correspond to the energy center surrounding the pineal gland, the nervous system (comprised of the brain and spinal cord), and the immune system as it relates to both. The pineal gland, which resembles a pine cone, is located deep in the brain where the right and left hemispheres connect, positioned close to the optical nerve. It was symbolically known by alchemists, the ancient Egyptians, and other spiritually minded groups as the "third eye," which is interesting when you see the deep connection between the pineal gland's function and what happens when we *see* light. The pineal gland's main role is the regulation of the sleep hormone melatonin, which impacts how well your immune system functions and your circadian rhythms (sense of day and night along with the shifting of light according to the seasons). During daylight hours, when we see light, secretions of melatonin are low; and during dark, night hours, secretions of melatonin are high. Sun exposure can also trigger the pineal gland along with an antidepressant effect that can boost cognitive abilities.

Caring for the pineal gland, and your immunity in general, with foods from this chapter, means you'll have better mental health and proper circadian rhythms. That means you'll feel alert throughout the day, get proper sleep, have an easier time waking up in the morning, and feel more "in the flow." A calm, balanced state of mind and healthy nervous system allow for deeper meditations, easy release of emotional upsets, and an ability to transcend day-to-day problems so you can focus on the big picture and pursue your main goals in life.

In alchemy, solidification is when all your holistic work starts to "gel," and you feel as if you have some traction physically, mentally, and emotionally. Think of that slang expression "that's solid!" and you'll get the sense. Achieving this level of balance is often thought to require a level of mastery of the three-fold alchemy principle—body, soul, and mind (spirit)—along with an acceptance of life's contradictions. But you don't have to be a master to start working on this energy center. Having regularly scheduled, calm-time rituals are key ways to support health in this area. The foods, soulful practices, and meditation in this chapter can become your end-of-day or postwork ritual to regroup, relax, and recharge your body so you can stave off illness and fatigue while accepting what life throws your way. The recipes in this chapter are lighter and more therapeutic in nature (and lower in calories), and can be used to rebalance after stressful days without overloading your digestive system.

Superfoods, Herbs, and Essential Oils for the Pineal Gland, Nervous System, and Immune System

MUSHROOMS: Both culinary mushrooms (such as shiitake and cremini) and medicinal mushrooms (such as reishi, chaga, and cordeceps) are über-superfoods for the nervous system. Culinary mushrooms are all very high in B vitamins, crucial for your brain and healthy nerves, specifically providing regeneration of nerve fibers and cells as well as better communication between neurons that allow the rest of your body to communicate info to the brain.

LEAFY GREENS: Leafy greens are bursting with vitamin C and iron, two synergistic nutrients that are important for the health of your pineal gland. Iron is a cofactor in the synthesis of serotonin, which your pineal gland needs to make melatonin. Vitamin C works as a superbooster for iron absorption, specifically when it comes to nonheme (plant) iron.

LAVENDER AND LAVENDER ESSENTIAL OIL: The top oil for nerve balance, lavender has a long been used as a tonic for the mind and well as an antibacterial, antimicrobial cleanser for the whole body. Lavender derives its name from the Latin *lavare*, meaning "to wash," and was prescribed orally by medieval physicians for treatment of epilepsy and migraine attacks. Modern medical studies (both in animals and humans) show that lavender oil produces significant antianxiety effects, making it a balm for your stressful day.

TURMERIC: The gold standard of healing, turmeric is featured in this chapter and throughout the book as it offers a multitude of health benefits and protection for the whole body. Turmeric is particularly helpful for the brain. Some smaller studies have recently shown that curcumin (the active compound in turmeric) is protective for the pineal gland since it can help the brain to detox from fluoride poisoning.

ECHINACEA: A beautiful drought-tolerant flowering plant in the daisy family, echinacea is often used as a home remedy for colds. A good amount of studies have shown that echinacea can help boost overall immunity with its protective, immunity-modulating compounds *E. purpurea* and *E. sanguinea* that are anti-inflammatory and antiviral.

FRANKINCENSE OIL: Made from the resin of the *Boswellia sacra* tree native to the Arabian Peninsula, frankincense is known for its role in sacred religious rituals and is used by energy healers to boost emotional well-being. It contains powerful detoxifying properties and is one of the top essential oils for cancer prevention.

LEMON BALM AND LEMON BALM OIL: For alchemists in the seventeenth century, lemon balm (*Melissa officinalis*) was one of the most prized herbs, considered an excellent way to calm and focus for meditation time as well as ease the stress of long days in the laboratory or working with ill patients. Some medical studies show that lemon balm does contain calming compounds that help ease stress.

This breakfast smoothie combines the jammy taste of blueberries with the chill factor of lavender, making it an ideal stressful Monday morning breakfast go-to. Blending in echinacea tea is also a great idea to boost immunity without changing the flavor. Allow the tea to cool completely before adding it to your blender, to avoid damaging any of the delicate nutrients from the other ingredients.

Lavender Blueberry Smoothie
WITH ECHINACEA TEA

SERVES 2

2 cups blueberries

⅔ cup protein powder or plain Greek yogurt

1 cup chilled echinacea tea

¼ cup almonds or walnuts

1 tablespoon honey or agave nectar, or 2 teaspoons stevia

2 teaspoon food-grade lavender flower buds

8 ice cubes

Place all the ingredients in a blend and process until smooth. Divide between two cups and serve immediately.

NOTE: To brew the tea, pour 1 cup of boiling water over one echinacea tea bag or 2 teaspoons of dried echinacea in an infuser. Steep for 10 minutes or longer. Let the tea cool completely before adding it to the smoothie.

per serving with protein powder and honey

321	calories
12 g (2 g)	fat (sat)
39 g	carbs
26 g	sugar
8 g	fiber
23 g	protein
85 mg	sodium

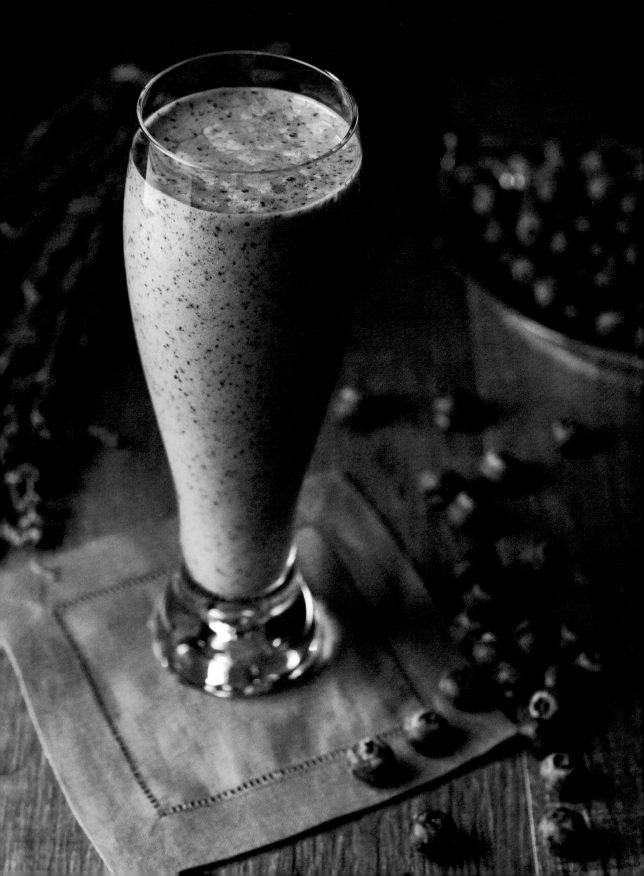

This refreshing drink calls to mind a beautiful sunrise because its brilliant orange is reminiscent of the sun in its glorious moment of transition. It's packed full of vitamin C for immunity and potent bioactive components from the turmeric, a superspice with over seven hundred medical studies behind it. A glass of this in the morning will give you a burst of energy for the day!

CARROT ORANGE TURMERIC
Sunburst Smoothie

SERVES 2

2 large carrots

1 orange, peeled

⅔ cup protein powder or Greek yogurt

½ cup unsweetened, shredded coconut

¼ cup almonds or walnuts

1 tablespoon honey or agave nectar, or 2 teaspoons stevia

1 tablespoon chopped fresh turmeric, or 1 teaspoon ground

8 ice cubes

Place the carrots, orange, protein powder, coconut, nuts, honey or agave, turmeric, and ice cubes in a blender. Blend until smooth. Divide between two cups and serve immediately.

per serving with Greek yogurt and honey
315 *calories*
18 g (8 g) *fat (sat)*
33 g *carbs*
23 g *sugar*
8 g *fiber*
13 g *protein*
87 mg *sodium*

This is a great "under the weather" beverage or a good substitution for your standard evening tea. When preparing it, be sure not to boil; rather, simmer the ingredients. Boiling medicinal foods can damage vital water-soluble nutrients, such as vitamin C, and other, even finer, cancer-fighting compounds.

HOT TURMERIC
Lemon Peel Tea

Peel the yellow zest from the lemon with a potato peeler, trying to avoid the white pith beneath. Place the zest and the remaining ingredients in a medium-size saucepan along with 1 quart of water. Bring to a simmer over medium heat, and cook for 2 to 3 minutes to allow the flavors to meld. Cover, remove from the heat, and steep for 5 minutes, then serve.

SERVES 2

1 lemon

2 tablespoons thinly sliced fresh turmeric, or 1 teaspoon ground

2 teaspoons honey or stevia

1 drop lemon or turmeric essential oil

per serving with honey

36	*calories*
0 g (0 g)	*fat (sat)*
9 g	*carbs*
7 g	*sugar*
1 g	*fiber*
0 g	*protein*
1 mg	*sodium*

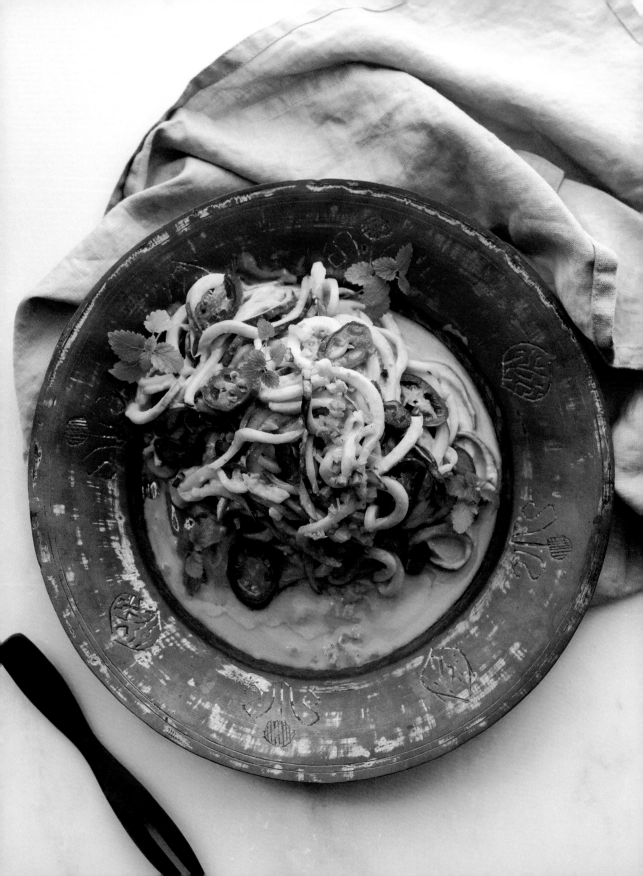

Craving takeout, but want to skip the unhealthy, tummy-bloating side effects? This dish is a playful nod to Chinese cold peanut noodles, with the same delectable sauce plus the healing addition of turmeric. Shop for this fresh, orange-fleshed root in your local organic market or even at the farmers' market. The outside is covered in a light brown skin, similar to ginger, but turmeric tends to be significantly smaller in size than ginger.

Cold Zucchini Noodles
WITH TURMERIC ROOT PEANUT SAUCE

SERVES 4

Prepare the sauce: Place the peanut butter, coconut milk, tamari, 1 tablespoon of the sesame oil or coconut oil, and the chili sauce in a blender along with ¼ cup of water. Blend until smooth and set aside.

Using a vegetable slicer or spiralizer, process the squash or zucchini into noodle shapes.

Heat the remaining 1 tablespoon of sesame oil in a large sauté pan over medium heat. Add the garlic, ginger, and turmeric and cook, stirring often, for 2 to 3 minutes, or until golden. Add the zucchini noodles and cook, tossing often, for 2 to 3 minutes more, or until the noodles are tender. Remove from the heat and let cool to room temperature, about 5 minutes. Toss with the peanut sauce and garnish with the cilantro, lemon balm or mint leaves, and jalapeño (if using). Serve immediately or transfer to a bowl and cover, then chill for at least 1 hour before serving.

⅓ cup peanut butter
or tahini paste

2 tablespoons canned
coconut milk

1 tablespoon low-sodium tamari

2 tablespoons sesame
or coconut oil

1 teaspoon hot chili sauce

4 large zucchini (2½ pounds)

2 garlic cloves, minced

1 tablespoon minced fresh ginger

1 tablespoon minced fresh
turmeric, or ½ teaspoon ground

8 cilantro sprigs

½ cup fresh lemon balm
or mint leaves

2 jalapeño peppers, thinly sliced
(optional)

---◇---
per serving
with peanut butter
230 *calories*
18 g (4 g) *fat (sat)*
12 g *carbs*
8 g *sugar*
4 g *fiber*
8 g *protein*
494 mg *sodium*
---◇---

213

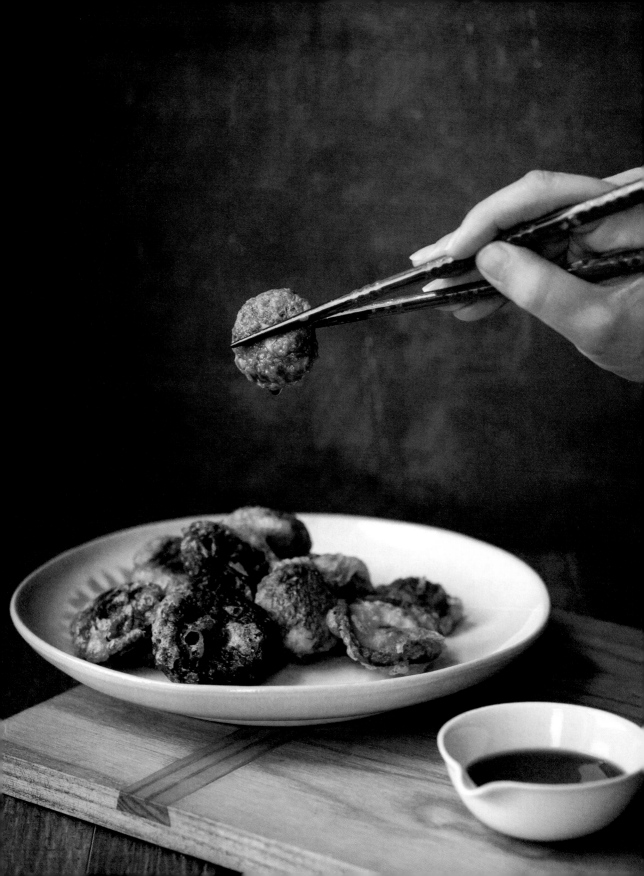

Tempura is a Japanese dish of vegetables or protein coated in a light batter and fried, often served as an appetizer. Fried food doesn't have to be bad for you if you use limited amounts of a good-quality fat, such as olive oil, as opposed to lower-grade oils, such as soybean or canola. Using leftover teas in recipes is a great way to get the power of medicinal foods into your meals. With a bitter, earthy flavor similar to green tea, reishi mushroom tea can be found in tea bags in health food stores or online.

Mushroom Tempura
WITH REISHI TEA GINGER DIPPING SAUCE

SERVES 4

Make the dipping sauce: Place the tea, tamari, ginger, and honey in a small bowl. Whisk well and set aside.

Line a rimmed baking sheet with paper towels. Remove and discard the stems from the mushrooms. Place the flour, cornstarch, ¾ cup of cold water, and ice cubes in a large bowl. Whisk to combine. Heat the oil in a small saucepan over medium heat.

Dip two of the shiitake caps into the flour mixture to evenly coat. Carefully drop the coated caps into the oil and cook for 3 to 4 minutes, or until the mushrooms start to brown, turning them with a fork about halfway through cooking. Don't move them early in the cooking process or they will stick to the pan. Transfer to the lined baking sheet and sprinkle with a pinch of the salt. Repeat with remaining mushroom caps and salt. Serve immediately with dipping sauce.

NOTE: To brew the tea, pour ½ cup boiling water over one reishi mushroom tea bag, cover, and steep for 10 minutes. If you have reishi in powder form rather than in tea bags, stir ½ teaspoon of powder into ½ cup of water and let it simmer for several minutes. Then cool.

½ cup cold reishi mushroom tea

4 tablespoons low-sodium tamari

1 tablespoon finely chopped fresh ginger

1 teaspoon honey or stevia

1 pound shiitake mushrooms

½ cup gluten-free multipurpose flour

2 teaspoons cornstarch

4 ice cubes

¼ cup olive or sesame oil

¼ teaspoon salt

— ◇ —
per serving
245 *calories*
14 g (2 g) *fat (sat)*
25 g *carbs*
5 g *sugar*
3 g *fiber*
6 g *protein*
864 mg *sodium*
— ◇ —

Have a sweet tooth after a hard workout? Try this in place of sugary sweet sports drinks that can perk you up momentarily but wreak havoc on your brain, slowing your ability to learn and damaging your memory. Brain-friendly lemon balm adds minty freshness to ruby red, sweet-tasting hibiscus that's naturally sugar-free.

LEMON BALM
Hibiscus Iced Tea

MAKES 1 QUART

1 orange

1 cup fresh lemon balm or mint leaves

2 hibiscus tea bags

2 teaspoons stevia (optional)

Peel the orange-colored zest from the orange with a potato peeler, trying to avoid the white pith beneath. Bring 1 quart of water to a boil in a medium-size saucepan. Turn off the heat. Add the orange peel, lemon balm, hibiscus tea bags, and stevia (if using). Cover and allow to cool. Transfer to an airtight container and keep refrigerated (leave the herbs in the tea to get more of their healing compounds).

per 8 ounce serving with stevia

79	*calories*
0 g (0 g)	*fat (sat)*
27 g	*carbs*
16 g	*sugar*
5 g	*fiber*
2 g	*protein*
8 mg	*sodium*

Lemon balm is one of the most prized herbs for healers and alchemists. Hildegard von Bingen, the twelfth-century nun, writer, philosopher, and herbalist, said, "Lemon balm contains within it the virtues of a dozen other plants." She used it in an elixir to prevent mental confusion and encouraged people to chew on lemon balm leaves to be more joyful. These light, balmy noodles are perfect for an easygoing spring party in your backyard. A strong finishing of freshly ground black pepper adds a bite and color to the dish's variety of soft, savory pastels.

LEMON BALM
Yellow Squash Noodles

Place the garlic, salt, and red pepper flakes (if using) in a food processor and pulse until finely chopped. Add the spinach, cilantro or basil, and lemon balm and pulse until the greens are finely chopped. Add the Parmesan and pulse until incorporated. Set aside.

Using a vegetable slicer or spiralizer, process the squash or zucchini into noodle shapes. Heat the olive oil in a large skillet over medium heat. Add the noodles and cook for 2 to 3 minutes, or until the noodles start to soften. Remove from the heat. Transfer the noodles to a large bowl and toss with the spinach mixture. Serve immediately.

SERVES 4

2 garlic cloves

½ teaspoon salt

½ teaspoon crushed red pepper flakes (optional)

2 cups baby spinach, kale, or watercress

1 cup fresh cilantro or basil

1 cup fresh lemon balm or mint leaves

¼ cup grated Parmesan cheese or walnuts

4 large yellow squash or zucchini

2 tablespoons olive oil

per serving
148 *calories*
9 g (2 g) *fat (sat)*
14 g *carbs*
7 g *sugar*
5 g *fiber*
7 g *protein*
399 mg *sodium*

Need a break from kale? Try watercress, a spicier leafy green in the cruciferous family that carries a similar nutritional profile to kale. Both pine nuts and hemp seeds, also called hemp hearts, can help bring on the "chill factor," since they are both incredibly high in magnesium. Magnesium is a supernutrient for the brain and the nervous system. It you're feeling on edge and extra-touchy, this may be a symptom of low levels of magnesium.

Mango Watercress Salad
WITH LEMON BALM PESTO DRESSING

SERVES 4

2 cups loosely packed fresh basil leaves

½ cup fresh lemon balm or mint leaves

1 garlic clove, cut into thirds

½ teaspoon salt

¼ teaspoon freshly ground black pepper

¼ cup pine nuts or shelled hemp seeds, plus 2 tablespoons for garnish

¼ cup grated Parmesan cheese (optional)

¼ cup extra-virgin olive oil

½ pound watercress

½ pound frisée or sliced radicchio

1 fresh mango, cubed, or 1½ cups frozen mango cubes, defrosted

1 red bell pepper, seeded and thinly sliced

Place the basil and lemon balm in a food processor and pulse ten to fifteen times, or until finely chopped. Add the garlic, salt, and black pepper and process again until the garlic is finely chopped. Add the ¼ cup pine nuts, Parmesan (if using), and olive oil and pulse again until a thick sauce forms. Add 2 tablespoons of warm water and pulse again to form a looser dressing.

Arrange the watercress, frisée or radicchio, mango, and bell pepper on a large platter. Drizzle with the dressing and serve immediately.

per serving
266 *calories*
20 g (3 g) *fat (sat)*
16 g *carbs*
9 g *sugar*
6 g *fiber*
9 g *protein*
420 mg *sodium*

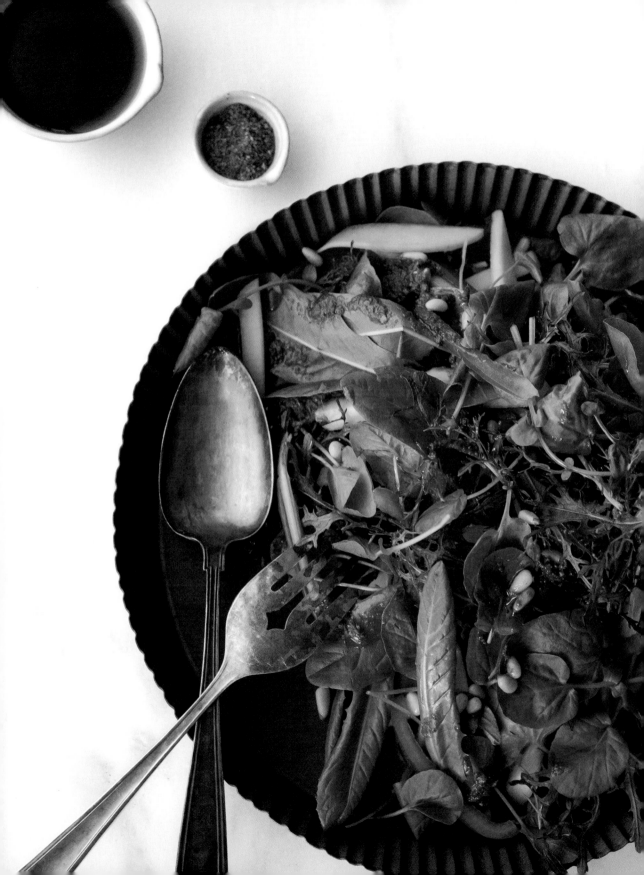

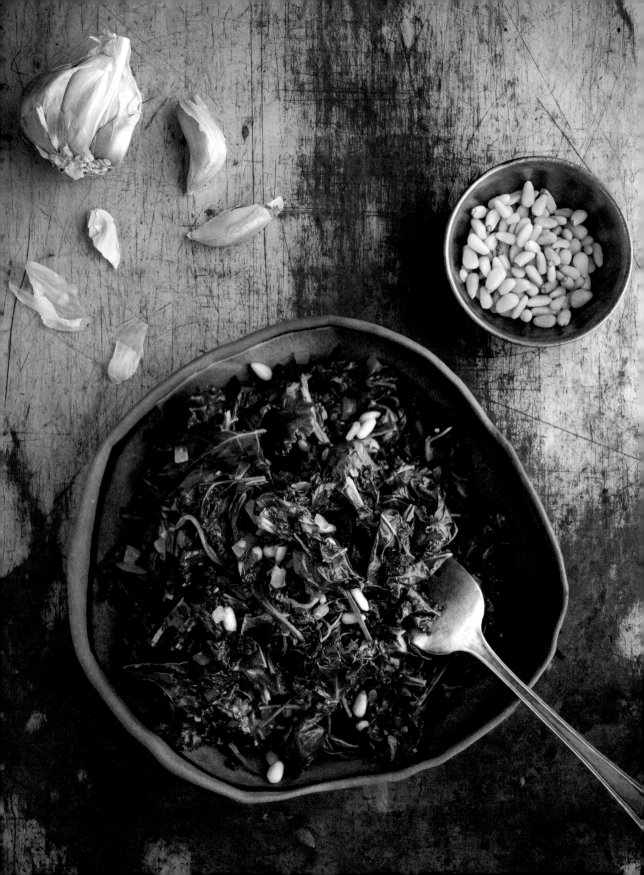

Make this simple side dish anytime you want to get more greens into your diet, fast. Pairing greens and nuts is an alchemical pairing for several reasons: it covers a broad range of healing nutrients for this energy center, including vitamin C and iron (from the greens), and a good dose of magnesium that's great for your brain and also helps calm your nervous system.

Sautéed Power Greens
WITH RAISINS AND PINE NUTS

Heat the oil in a large skillet over medium heat and add the onion or shallots and garlic. Sprinkle with the salt and pepper. Cook, stirring occasionally, for 6 to 8 minutes, or until the onion starts to brown. Working in batches, add the greens, tossing them with the onion mixture and cooking until the greens wilt, about 2 minutes. Transfer the wilted greens to a platter and repeat remaining greens.

Once all the greens are wilted, top them with the pine nuts and raisins and serve.

SERVES 4

2 tablespoons olive oil

½ red onion or 1 shallot, chopped

4 garlic cloves, minced

½ teaspoon salt

½ teaspoon freshly ground black pepper

1 pound mixed power greens

¼ cup pine nuts

½ cups regular or golden raisins

---

per serving
186 *calories*
12 g (4 g) *fat (sat)*
17 g *carbs*
11 g *sugar*
3 g *fiber*
3 g *protein*
215 mg *sodium*

Topical Magnesium
Magnesium, necessary for nerve and brain function, as well as general disease prevention, is a vital mineral that most people are deficient in and they don't even know it. Although you'll find it in high quantities in both nuts and seeds, magnesium can also be absorbed through the skin. Try Epsom salts, mixed with your favorite herbs or essential oil, for a mineral-rich bath or treat yourself to magnesium creams and oil sprays. Note: These creams and sprays do sting slightly upon first application, which is normal.

221

This recipe features the superfood kale, which is rich in vitamin K and comes in a variety of textures and colors at most grocery stores and markets. Combine it with crunchy roasted pumpkin seeds, creamy avocado, and a sweet and spicy dressing to add a unique and memorable glaze to these healthy leaves.

Mixed Power Greens Salad
WITH MAPLE TURMERIC DRESSING

SERVES 4

¼ cup pumpkin seeds

¼ cup pure maple syrup

¼ cup olive oil

1 tablespoon cider vinegar

1 teaspoon ground turmeric

½ teaspoon salt

½ teaspoon freshly ground black pepper

½ pound baby spinach

½ pound kale

1 avocado, pitted, peeled, and thinly sliced

Preheat an oven or toaster oven to 300°F. Place the pumpkin seeds on a dry sheet pan and roast for 10 to 12 minutes, or until they start to brown. Set aside to cool.

Place the maple syrup, olive oil, vinegar, turmeric, salt, and pepper in a large bowl. Whisk well to combine. Add the greens and toss well. Top with the avocado and sprinkle with the pumpkin seeds. Serve immediately.

per serving
297 *calories*
23 g (3 g) *fat (sat)*
20 g *carbs*
12 g *sugar*
5 g *fiber*
6 g *protein*
363 mg *sodium*

Stroganoff, a classic beef dish with a rich creamy sauce, is reimagined using a top food for this energy center—mushrooms! Any mushrooms from button to cremini, and even wild mushrooms, will work in this dish, but if you want more medicinal compounds in your meal, use shiitake.

SAGE-SMOKED
Mushroom Stroganoff

SERVES 4

Arrange the mushrooms on a wire cooling rack, gathering them in a small pile in the center of the rack. Place the sage on a baking sheet. In a well-ventilated kitchen, light the sage with matches and allow the flame to go out so the sage smolders. Place the rack of mushrooms directly over the smoldering sage, and place a large metal bowl over the mushrooms, but still allowing air underneath so that the sage continues to smoke. Allow them to smoke for 10 to 15 minutes, or until the sage stops smoking. Slice the mushrooms and set aside.

Heat 2 tablespoons of the oil in a large skillet over medium heat. Add the onion, garlic, salt, and pepper cook for 7 to 8 minutes, or until the onion is tender and browned. Add the mushrooms, cover, and cook for 3 to 4 minutes more, or until the mushrooms have released their liquid and are tender.

Sprinkle the mushrooms with the flour, toss well, and cook for 1 minute more. Add the stock and wine (if using) and cook, stirring continuously, for 1 minute. Turn off the heat and allow to cool for a few minutes while you prepare the garnish.

Heat the remaining tablespoon of oil in a small skillet and add the sage. Fry for 1 minute, or until crisp, then turn off the heat. Stir in the coconut cream. Spoon the mushroom mixture over the cooked grains and garnish with the sage mixture. Serve immediately.

1 pound mushrooms, any variety

1 cup dried sage

3 tablespoons olive oil

1 onion, thinly sliced

2 garlic cloves, minced

½ teaspoon salt

½ teaspoon freshly ground black pepper

2 tablespoons gluten-free multipurpose flour

½ cup vegetable stock

½ cup white wine, or an additional ½ cup stock

½ cup fresh sage leaves

¼ cup coconut cream or sour cream

1 cup uncooked quinoa or millet, cooked according to the package instructions

---◇---

per serving
372 *calories*
16 g (4 g) *fat (sat)*
41 g *carbs*
0 g *sugar*
5 g *fiber*
11 g *protein*
485 mg *sodium*

---◇---

223

This fruit salad is summer in a bowl, full of natural vibrant colors and flavors. Lemon balm is great for stress management or any moment when you need to calm your mind. Make this dish and you'll be kicking back enjoying the good life in no time!

LEMON BALM
Fruit Salad

SERVES 8

2 cups strawberries, hulled

2 cups assorted berries, such as blueberries, raspberries, and blackberries

1 small watermelon, thinly sliced or cubed

½ cup fresh lemon balm leaves, torn

Edible flowers (optional)

2 tablespoons elderberry or pure maple syrup

Arrange the strawberries, other berries, and watermelon on a platter or in a large bowl. Sprinkle the fruit with lemon balm and edible flowers (if using). Drizzle with the elderberry syrup and serve.

per serving
216 *calories*
1 g (0 g) *fat (sat)*
54 g *carbs*
43 g *sugar*
4 g *fiber*
4 g *protein*
7 mg *sodium*

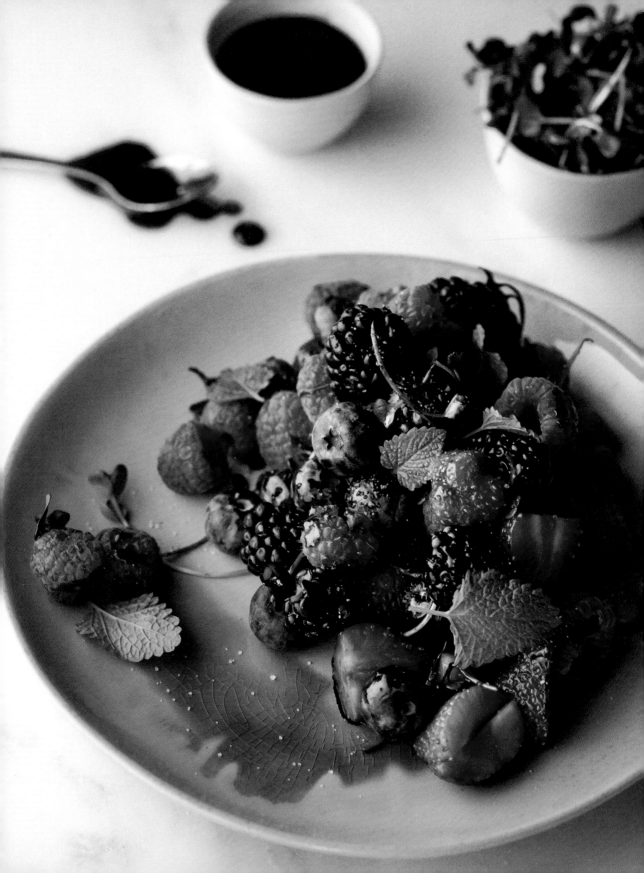

Chilled soups are a great way to "chill out" on a hot day, and this dish does double duty since it contains nutrients that also calm the nervous system—vitamin C with iron. It couldn't be easier to make. A quick toss in the blender and you have a delicious, unusual soup, rich in leafy green goodness. You can eat it hot or cooled.

CHILLED GREEN GRAPE
Spinach Soup

SERVES 4

3 cups green grapes

6 cups baby spinach

2 cups vegetable stock

½ cup fresh basil leaves

⅓ cup hazelnuts

4 scallions, chopped (optional)

1 red bell pepper, seeded and chopped

Place the grapes, baby spinach, stock, basil, and hazelnuts in a blender and process until smooth. Top with the chopped scallions (if using) and bell pepper. Serve immediately. Alternatively, to serve heated, transfer to a small saucepan and warm over low heat for 4 to 5 minutes.

per serving
236 *calories*
12 g (1 g) *fat (sat)*
30 g *carbs*
20 g *sugar*
6 g *fiber*
7 g *protein*
501 mg *sodium*

Asian dishes get their crave-worthy umami flavor from rich-tasting ingredients, such as mushrooms, sesame, and tamari. Tamari is a gluten-free, fermented sauce made from soybeans and is similar in flavor to soy sauce. You can substitute it one for one in any recipe calling for soy sauce. Shiitake mushrooms not only bring their unique flavor to the dish but eight essential amino acids, along with potent antimicrobial and antitumor properties.

Rainbow Buddha Bowl
WITH CREAMY SESAME SHIITAKE DRESSING

Prepare the dressing: Heat the sesame oil in a small skillet over medium heat. Add the mushrooms, garlic salt, and pepper. Cook, stirring often, for 4 to 5 minutes, or until the mushrooms start to soften. Turn off the heat. Transfer to a bowl along with the mayonnaise, vinegar, tamari, garlic, sesame seeds, and 2 tablespoons of warm water. Stir well.

Place the kale, carrots, avocado, tomatoes, and cucumber in a large bowl. Drizzle with the dressing and toss well. Serve immediately.

SERVES 4

2 tablespoons sesame oil

8 ounces shiitake mushrooms, stems discarded, chopped

½ teaspoon garlic salt

¼ teaspoon freshly ground black pepper

¼ cup mayonnaise or vegan mayonnaise

2 tablespoons cider vinegar

2 tablespoons low-sodium tamari

1 garlic clove, minced

1 tablespoon toasted sesame seeds

½ pound baby kale

2 carrots, peeled and cut into ribbons or thinly sliced

1 avocado, pitted, peeled, and sliced

½ pound cherry tomatoes, quartered

1 small cucumber, diced

---

2 cups vegetables plus ⅓ cup dressing
307 *calories*
24 g (3 g) *fat (sat)*
22 g *carbs*
7 g *sugar*
7 g *fiber*
6 g *protein*
651 mg *sodium*

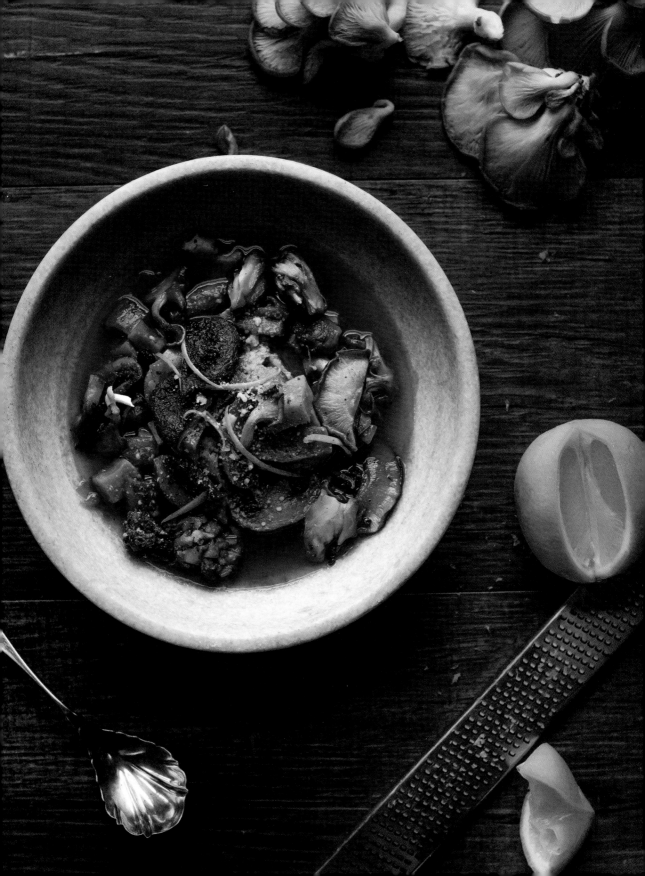

What's more comforting than a bowl of hot soup on a cold day, especially when it's accented by a mild peppery spice like paprika? This recipe combines the earthy flavors of mushrooms with the sweetness of onion and corn for a soul-nourishing bowl of goodness. Research has suggested that paprika may even have anticancer and antiaging properties. Digesting it with fat allows the body to incorporate its benefits and seal in its effects.

RUSTIC PAPRIKA-SPIKED
Mushroom Soup

Place the butter in a large stockpot and melt over medium heat. Add the mushrooms, onion, salt, and pepper. Cook, stirring occasionally, for 5 to 7 minutes, or until the onion starts to soften and the mushrooms give off their liquid. Add the paprika and stir to coat the vegetables. Add the potatoes and stock. Bring to a boil, then immediately lower the heat to a simmer. Cover and cook for 25 to 30 minutes, or until the potatoes are fork-tender. Add the corn and cook for 4 minutes more.

Divide the soup among four bowls and sprinkle with the Parmesan (if using), parsley, and orange zest. Serve immediately.

2 tablespoons unsalted grass-fed butter or olive oil

1 pound mushrooms, such as shiitake or cremini

1 medium-size sweet onion, chopped

½ teaspoon salt

¼ teaspoon freshly ground black pepper

2 tablespoons mild paprika

½ pound baby potatoes, such as red bliss or purple Peruvian, diced

1 quart vegetable stock

2 cups corn kernels

½ cup grated Parmesan cheese or nutritional yeast (optional)

½ cup chopped fresh parsley or cilantro

2 teaspoons orange or lemon zest

---

per serving

259	calories
10 g (6 g)	fat (sat)
37 g	carbs
10 g	sugar
6 g	fiber
11 g	protein
623 mg	sodium

229

Chocolate, turmeric, and black pepper are an alchemy power trio. Turmeric absorbs better with the addition of a healthy fat from chocolate and piperine, a compound in black pepper that keeps turmeric in your body longer for better uptake. If you want to boost your uptake further, pair these truffles with a cup of warm tea or milk, since studies show that heat also improves how well we can absorb turmeric.

TURMERIC CHOCOLATE
Hemp Truffles

MAKES 32 TRUFFLES

1 cup almonds

¼ cup hemp seeds

½ cup heavy cream or coconut cream

1 teaspoon ground turmeric

¼ teaspoon freshly ground black pepper

8 ounces 70% cocoa bittersweet chocolate, chopped

4 teaspoons stevia

½ teaspoon pure vanilla extract

2 tablespoons unsweetened cocoa powder

Place the almonds and hemp seeds in a food processor and finely chop. Bring the cream, turmeric, and pepper to a boil in a small saucepan over medium-high heat. Remove from the heat and add the chocolate, stevia, and vanilla. Let sit for 2 to 3 minutes, then whisk until smooth. Stir in the almond mixture. Let cool to room temperature, then refrigerate, uncovered, until the mixture is firm, about 1 hour.

Spoon mounds (1 heaping teaspoon each) of the chilled chocolate mixture onto a large plate or sheet pan lined with parchment or waxed paper. Place the pan in the refrigerator to chill for 15 minutes.

Roll the mounds into smooth balls. Place the cocoa powder on a plate. Roll the balls in the cocoa and transfer to a small tray. Chill until set, about 30 minutes. Serve immediately or store, refrigerated, in an airtight container for up to 2 weeks.

	2 truffles
164	calories
14 g (6 g)	fat (sat)
10 g	carbs
4 g	sugar
3 g	fiber
5 g	protein
1 mg	sodium

THE SUPERFOOD ALCHEMY COOKBOOK

Honey can be used both as a sweetener and as a salve. Throughout ancient history, honey was used for accelerating wound healing in ulcers, infected wounds, and kitchen or laboratory burns for the alchemist. It appears in this chapter as an immunity-boosting food since honey has been reported to have an inhibitory effect on around sixty species of bacteria, including aerobes and anaerobes.

Herb-Infused Honey

Place the honey in a small, airtight container along with your herb of choice. Stir well and cover. Store in a dark, cool cabinet for at least 3 days before using, to allow the flavors to meld.

½ cup honey, any variety

4 sprigs dried food-grade lavender, rosemary, thyme, or oregano

1 tablespoon
68 *calories*
0 g (0 g) *fat (sat)*
18 g *carbs*
17 g *sugar*
0 g *fiber*
0 g *protein*
1 mg *sodium*

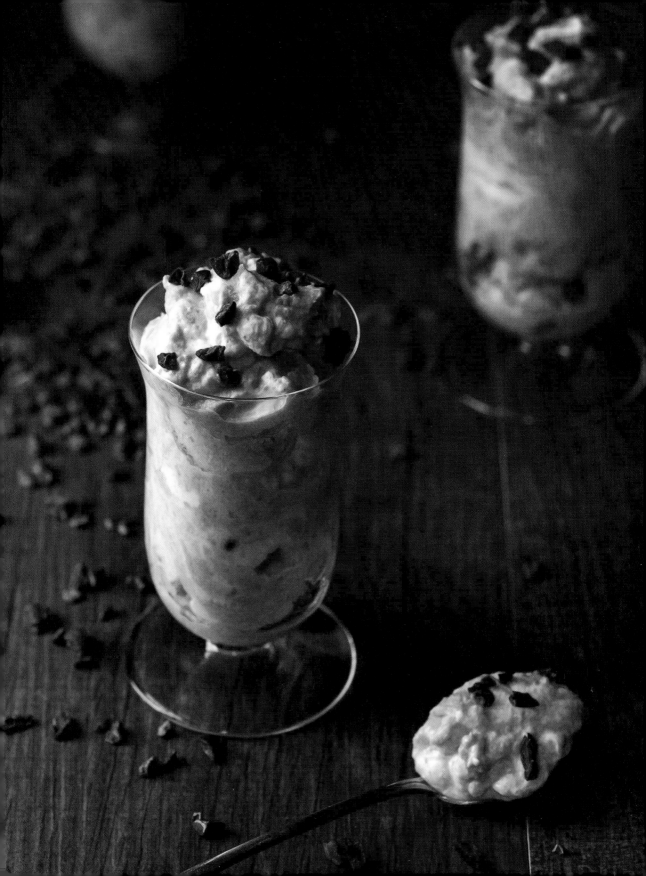

Nutmeg and cacao are delicious superfoods for your brain, rich in neuron-healing antioxidants called flavonols that give chocolate its earthy flavor. Fatty cream—dairy or coconut—serves two purposes: adding a fluffy texture while aiding in the uptake of such nutrients as the beta-carotene found in the pumpkin.

NUTMEG CACAO NIB
Pumpkin Mousse

SERVES 8

Place the pumpkin, ¼ cup of the cacao nibs, the honey or stevia, and the vanilla in a large bowl and mix well to combine. Set aside.

If using the heavy cream, place it in a large bowl. Using an electric mixer, beat the cream on high speed for 3 to 4 minutes, or until the mixture is light, thick, and fluffy and clings to the sides of the bowl when tipped. Add half the whipped heavy cream or the whipped coconut topping to the pumpkin mixture, fold lightly to incorporate, and transfer to eight parfait glasses.

Top with the remaining whipped cream or whipped coconut topping and garnish with remaining ¼ cup of cacao nibs. Serve immediately or chill for up to 4 hours, until ready to serve.

1 (15-ounce) can pure pumpkin puree

½ cup cacao nibs

¼ cup honey, or 2 tablespoons stevia

1 tablespoon pure vanilla extract

1 cup chilled heavy cream, or 2 cups whipped coconut topping

1 teaspoon freshly ground nutmeg

per serving
229 *calories*
17 g (11 g) *fat (sat)*
17 g *carbs*
11 g *sugar*
4 g *fiber*
2 g *protein*
15 mg *sodium*

Essential Oil Preparations and Rituals for Solidification

DIFFUSER OIL BLEND TO PROMOTE SLEEP

One of the primary reasons you should be using essential oils, if you aren't already, is to benefit from their incredible soothing, nerve-balancing properties. If you only buy one, choose lavender, and consider it your go-to oil! Dab a drop of lavender oil directly on your wrists or temples, or enjoy lavender oil in an essential oil diffuser to infuse your space with healing scent. Or use this blend with cedarwood and frankincense oils.

3 drops lavender essential oil

2 drops cedarwood essential oil

2 drops frankincense essential oil

Fill your essential oil diffuser with water according to the diffuser instructions. Add the oils and turn on the mister.

SLEEPYTIME FOOT SERUM

My dear friend and fellow chef/herbalist Meredith Chartier gave me this recipe, which I adapted to my own tastes. This ritual combines soothing essential oils and self-massage for an evening-time practice to help you get restful sleep—a key component of caring for the nervous system and immune system that helps the pineal gland do its job. If you like, for an extra immunity and relaxation boost, start the ritual by drinking a hot cup of nettle tea (page 22). Apply the serum by massaging a few drops into the soles of your feet, and put on thick comfortable socks. Add a soft silk sleep mask to shut out light for a deeper, more restful sleep.

MAKES 2 OUNCES

2 tablespoons almond or jojoba oil

10 drops vetiver essential oil

5 drops lavender essential oil

5 drops cedarwood essential oil

2 drops frankincense essential oil

2 drops lemon balm essential oil

Place the almond oil, vetiver, lavender, cedarwood, frankincense, and lemon balm oil in a 2-ounce dropper bottle or any small glass container with a lid. Close the bottle and shake gently to combine. Before bedtime, rub two or three drops on the sole of each foot, pulling on socks if desired.

LAVENDER LINEN SPRAY

Use this refreshing spray to add a subtle scent to your linens, robe, or eye pillow before sleep or meditation. Lavender has soothing properties and works well alongside other, woodier scents; try using rose-scented witch hazel. Or add a few drops of cedarwood for a spalike essence, or orange or lemon for added freshness.

MAKES 4 OUNCES

2 tablespoons unscented witch hazel

10 drops lavender essential oil

Place the witch hazel and essential oil in the spray bottle and close the top. Shake well to combine. Add ⅓ cup of water and shake again. Use for linens or as an air freshener.

STAUNCH A NOSEBLEED

Place a drop of lavender oil on a tissue and wrap it around one ice cube. Find a comfortable place where you can recline. Gently press the prepared tissue against the nostrils, breathing in and out slowly for 1 to 2 minutes until nose bleed subsides.

LAVENDER HEADACHE BALM

This delicious-smelling headache balm contains peppermint, a well-known analgesic (pain remedy). This is a helpful travel and work companion with the same soothing creamy consistency as lip balm. Keep it in your carry-on or work bag.

MAKES 4

4 (10 ml) lip balm containers

3 tablespoons coconut or jojoba oil

2 tablespoons beeswax pellets

10 drops lavender essential oil

10 drops peppermint essential oil

5 drops frankincense essential oil

Set out the lip balm containers on a counter and remove the lids. Place the oil and beeswax pellets in a small saucepan over low heat. Stirring constantly, heat for 3 to 4 minutes, or until the pellets melt. Turn off the heat and add the essential oils, stirring once or twice to combine. Transfer to a measuring cup with a spout and immediately pour into the lip balm containers.

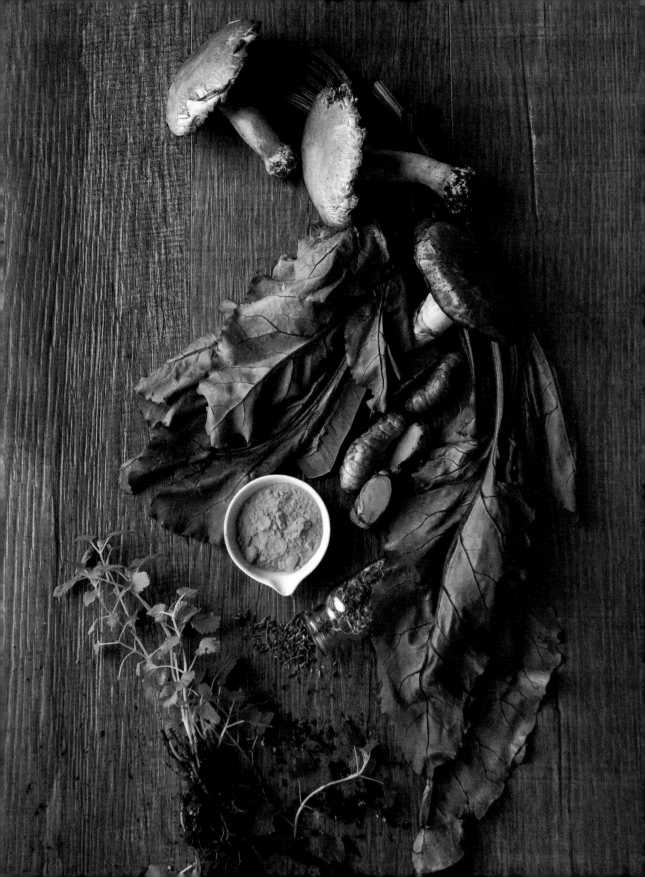

Meditation to Calm the Nerves and Promote Relaxation

GO WITH THE FLOW— UNDERSTANDING BRAINWAVES

Brain waves, or the electrical activity emanating from the brain, have everything to do with our state of consciousness. Meditation works by triggering different brain wave states, so understanding the different waves, and feeling them within yourself, can greatly improve your meditation practice.

BETA: The fastest waves, 15 to 40 cycles a minute. The brain is alert or aroused. Beta waves happen throughout the day as we interact with people and solve problems.

ALPHA: A nonaroused yet still active state, 9 to 14 cycles a minute. The state of rest after a more intense beta activity (think: a lunch break after a challenging meeting).

THETA: A slower, dreaming or daydreaming state, between 5 and 8 cycles a minute. Can allow for the feeling of flow where ideas or creative intuition will blossom. When we sleep, we experience a mix of theta and delta waves.

DELTA: The slowest wave, 1.4 to 4 cycles per minute. Experienced during deep, dreamless sleep, typically the type of non-REM sleep state that triggers healing in the body.

Searching for Stars

This nondirective meditation is intended to help you intensely concentrate, then release, promoting relaxation. Do this meditation in a dark room, preferably with a sleep mask. Start by closing your eyes. If it helps you, feel free to listen to calming music containing binaural beats without words. If any thoughts pop into your head, treat them as passing clouds: you may notice them, but do not engage or develop the thoughts further. After a time, you will notice that thoughts will come and go.

Healing Stone Therapy
Selenite, Herkimer diamond, and kyanite are all healing crystals for this area. While practicing any of the meditations featured in this book, you can rest one of these crystals against the top of your head. Earrings are a great option to wear any of these crystals.

With your eyes continually closed, look straight ahead as if peering into the dark night sky, looking for a star on a cloudy evening. Stay focused and concentrated until your eyes begin to release and you lose vision focus. If thoughts start to form, begin again and repeat until you are relaxed and in dark silence. The goal is to sit with no thoughts, sounds, or physical sensations.

Over time, you will become aware of going from a beta state to theta (you may begin to lucid dream). You can pull your mind away from the theta state with a little concentration and be back in the quiet of a silent beta, or allow yourself to continue dreaming in theta, and fall into deeper sleep.

MORE ON MEDITATION

Think of meditation as medicine and nourishment for your mind, since it's the active "thinking" consciousness that can create a sense of wellness in the body—just based on what you think and how often. Continuous stressful or negative thoughts paired with long work hours and little sleep can severely impact health: when stress hormones, such as cortisol, are released too often, it can cause low-grade inflammation that later may turn into auto-immune illness or organ issues. (This is one of the reasons stress is listed by doctors as the #1 cause of disease.) Meditation is hugely beneficial for emotional health, instilling a sense of well-being and self-reliance. Controlling thoughts and focusing the mind is a free, easy, safe, and superavailable treatment for stress that you can do in just ten minutes a day.

Studies have also shown that regular meditation and mindfulness practices have a physical effect on your brain, much like exercise for your body. As you age, your brain shrinks, specifically your frontal cortex consisting of gray matter. But you can slow the aging process of your brain with mediation, since people in their fifties who meditate regularly have the same mass of grey matter compared to their twenty-five-year-old counterparts. One study also showed that mediating for a period of just eight weeks resulted in "thicker brain mass" in four different regions.

Concentrative and Nondirective Meditation

Meditations typically fall into two categories, concentrative and nondirective. Concentrative requires concentrating your mind on something, whether it is a mantra or saying or word, such as the meditations from previous chapters. Nondirective is a form of meditation where you don't concentrate at all, but allow your mind to empty and your body to relax into a state of peace. You will find both types of meditation in this book, but nondirective is the most challenging, and unfortunately the reason why people quit meditation or get frustrated so fast when they try to learn this style first. If you are struggling to turn off your active brain, you're not alone! Listening to a track of music, rain, or waves with binaural beats added (a 4.5 beats-per-second frequency, which mimics the theta brainwave state—see page 237), can help lull you into a deeper state. Or you may wish to start with a concentrative meditation first, and then spend five minutes on nondirective at the end of your practice.

Meditation Preparation

Before you begin, follow these easy preparations to get the most out of your mediation time. Create a small collection of meditation music that you can use each time you meditate. Using the same familiar songs can help calm the mind quickly, like a musical trigger to help get you into the flow right away. The more familiar the song, the less distracting as well. Find a quiet, dark room; light can be distracting. You can start in a room with some natural light with the shades pulled down. As you advance, you can find a fully dark room and/or use a sleep mask.

As you progress through the stages of meditation, you may have an experience where you cease to feel your body but are still conscious, which can be disorienting, especially for beginners. This protective, shielding visualization helps create a "hermetic seal" in the mind. It can help you hold on to a sense of calm and safety to meditate more deeply. (If you already have a set preparation for mediation, you can continue to use it, and simply add this additional protective practice before you begin.)

PROTECTIVE VISUALIZATION

Close your eyes. Take a deep breath, hold it for a count of four, then slowly let it out to a count of four. Check in with your body to see where there is tension. Imagine there is a small grate over the area where the tension is, and breathe outside air in through the grate, while you release the muscles in that area. Repeat in all the areas that have tension, spending 3 to 4 minutes on this exercise. Next, visualize a stream of gold light starting to grow around you head, continuing to breathe in and out to a count of four. Imagine the bright gold light pouring in a thick stream down the front of your body from your head to toes, encompassing your feet and continuing past your feet up around your legs and back, finally reaching your head to connect at the top, creating a perfect oval circuit. Imagine this circuit starting to fan out across the front and back of your body, forming a perfect oval capsule around your body. Imagine the light capsule hardening like a shell, but retaining its golden gleam. Visualize this shell protecting and standing between you and outside energies and disturbances.

WORKING WITH CRYSTALS

Crystals and minerals hold a special place in the advanced alchemist laboratory, but even a newbie can enjoy the beauty of crystals by pairing them with various energy centers. Crystals in alchemy are meant to reinforce the energy of the center or amplify intention; each chapter lists specific crystals for that energy center. To use crystals during your meditations, recline on a comfortable surface, such as your bed or couch, before beginning the mediation. Place the appropriate crystal over the energy center, allow it to rest there during the meditation.

Crystal Elixirs

Making a crystal elixir is an easy way to charge your water or wine with the vibrations of your favorite healing stones. First, select crystals from your collection that are nontoxic. Any of the quartz crystals, such as rose and white quartz, amethyst, and carnelian, should be safe. Double check for potential toxic components in your elixirs if you plan on drinking them and using them on your body. Wash the stones with soap and hot water and rinse well under hot water. Place the crystals in an airtight glass jar and cover with filtered or distilled water. Rest the jar on the countertop at least three days, then try these easy ways to enjoy the elixir:

Spray it into your aura or add a drop of rose oil for a simple face atomizer.

Add it to your bath water along with any other desired bath products.

Add a few drops of your favorite essential oils and use as a room spray.

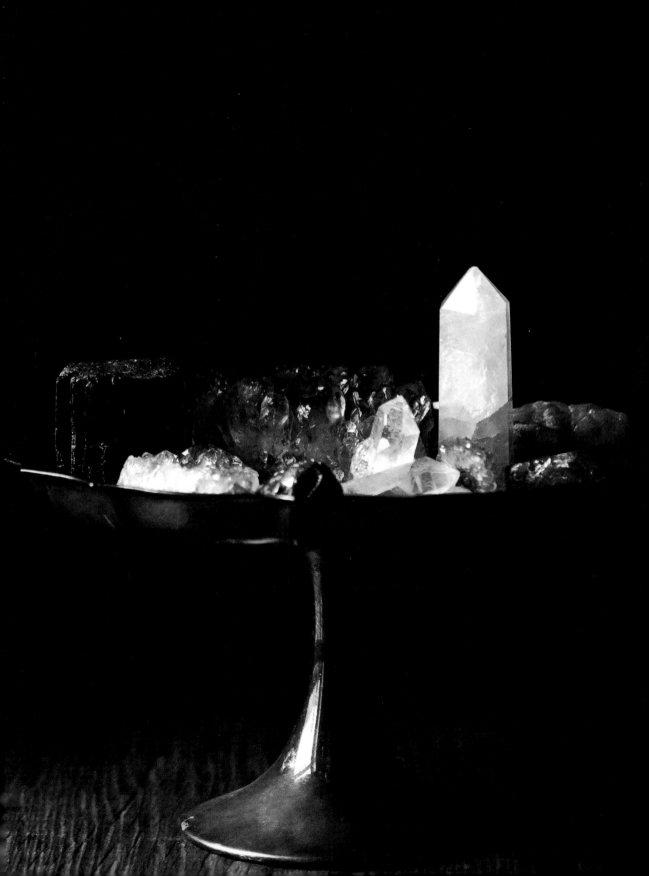

RECIPE INDEX

243

BIBLIOGRAPHY

Introduction

Campbell, A. W. "Autoimmunity and the Gut." *Autoimmune Diseases* 2014 (2014): 152428. doi:10.1155/2014/152428.

Clark, C. "Use Cast Iron Cookware as an Iron Deficiency Treatment." *University Health News Daily*, February 8, 2018. https://universityhealthnews.com/daily/energy/use-cast-iron-cookware-as-an-iron-deficiency-treatment.

"Meditation: In Depth." National Center for Complementary and Integrative Health (NCCIH), US Department of Health & Human Services, September 7, 2017. https://nccih.nih.gov/health/meditation/overview.htm.

Samsel, A., and S. Seneff. "Glyphosate, Pathways to Modern Diseases II: Celiac Sprue and Gluten Intolerance." *Interdisciplinary Toxicology* 6, no. 4 (2013): 159–184.

Chapter 1

Biehl, M., et al. "Evaluation of a Superactivated Charcoal Paste and Detergent and Water in Prevention of T-2 Toxin-Induced Local Cutaneous Effects in Topically Exposed Swine." *Toxicological Sciences* 13, no. 3 (October 1, 1989): 523–532.

Cheaha, D., et al. "Modification of Sleep-Waking and Electroencephalogram Induced by Vetiver Essential Oil Inhalation." *Journal of Intercultural Ethnopharmacology* 5, no. 1 (2016): 72–78.

Chiang, H. M., et al. "Rhodiola Plants: Chemistry and Biological Activity." *Journal of Food and Drug Analysis* 23, no. 3 (2015): 359–369.

Clifford, T., et al. "The Potential Benefits of Red Beetroot Supplementation in Health and Disease." *Nutrients* 7, no. 4 (2015): 2801–2822.

Gladding, R. "This Is Your Brain on Meditation." *Psychology Today* [blog], May 22, 2013. http://www.psychologytoday.com/us/blog/use-your-mind-change-your-brain/201305/is-your-brain-meditation.

Jacob, R., et al. "Neuroprotective Effect of *Rhodiola Rosea* Linn Against MPTP Induced Cognitive Impairment and Oxidative Stress." *Annals of Neurosciences* 20, no. 2 (2013): 47–51. PubMed Central, https://www.ncbi.nlm.nih.gov/pmc/articles/PMC4117113.

Janssens, P., et al. "Acute Effects of Capsaicin on Energy Expenditure and Fat Oxidation in Negative Energy Balance." *PLoS ONE* 8, no. 7 (2013): e67786. PubMed Central, https://www.ncbi.nlm.nih.gov/pubmed/23844093.

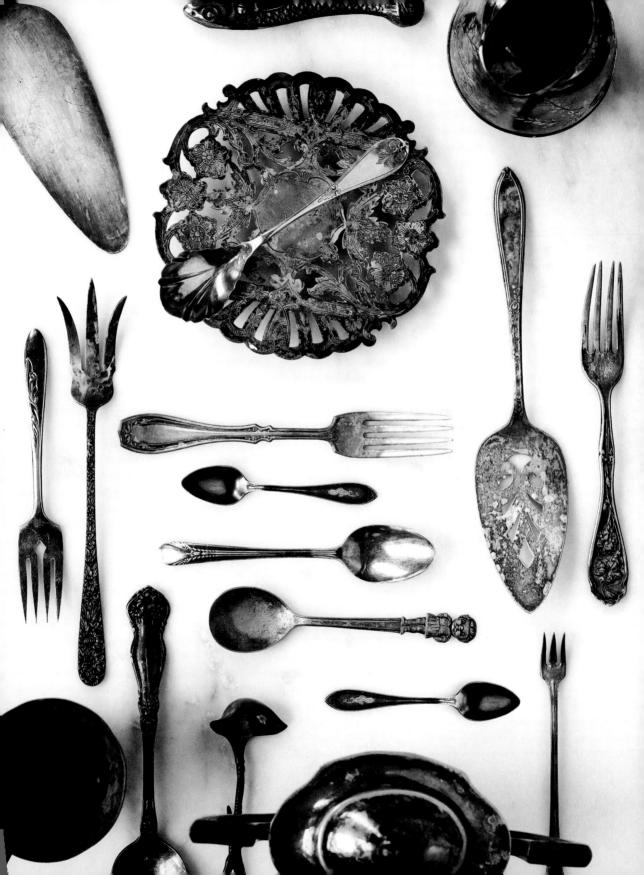

McCarty, M. F., et al. "Capsaicin May Have Important Potential for Promoting Vascular and Metabolic Health." *Open Heart* (2015); 2:e000262. doi: 10.1136/openhrt-2015-000262.

Surh, Y.-J. "More Than Spice: Capsaicin in Hot Chili Peppers Makes Tumor Cells Commit Suicide." *JNCI: Journal of the National Cancer Institute* 94, no. 17 (September 4, 2002): 1263–1265.

Chapter 2

Axe, J. "3 Steps to Heal Adrenal Fatigue Naturally." Dr. Axe. No date. https://draxe.com/3-steps-to-heal-adrenal-fatigue.

Bode, A. M., and Z. Dong. "The Amazing and Mighty Ginger." In *Herbal Medicine: Biomolecular and Clinical Aspects*, edited by I. F. F. Benzie and S. Wachtel-Galor. 2nd ed. Boca Raton, FL: CRC Press/Taylor & Francis, 2011.

Johnson, R. J., et al. "Uric Acid and Chronic Kidney Disease: Which Is Chasing Which?" *Nephrology, Dialysis, Transplantation* 28, no. 9 (September 2013): 2221–2228. doi: 10.1093/ndt/gft029. Epub March 29, 2013.

"Kidneys and Diabetes." Diabetes.co.uk. https:// diabetes.co.uk/body/kidneys.html.

Lila, M. A. "Anthocyanins and Human Health: An in Vitro Investigative Approach." *Journal of Biomedicine and Biotechnology* 2004, no. 5 (2004): 306–313. doi:10.1155/S111072430440401X.

Mayo Clinic Staff. "Dietary Fiber: Essential for a Healthy Diet." Mayo Foundation for Medical Education and Research. September 22, 2015. https://www.mayoclinic.org.

McCarty, M. F., J. J. DiNicolantonio, and J. H. O'Keefe. "Capsaicin May Have Important Potential for Promoting Vascular and Metabolic Health." *Open Heart* 2 (2015): e000262.

Nair, A. R., et al. "A Blueberry-Enriched Diet Improves Renal Function and Reduces Oxidative Stress in Metabolic Syndrome Animals: Potential Mechanism of TLR4-MAPK Signaling Pathway." *PLoS ONE* 9, no. 11 (2014): e111976.

Chapter 3

Ahn, T.-B., and B. S. Jeon. "The Role of Quercetin on the Survival of Neuron-Like PC12 Cells and the Expression of α-synuclein." *Neural Regeneration Research* 10, no. 7 (2015): 1113–1119.

Ash, M. "Vitamin A: The Key to a Tolerant Immune System?" Clinical Education, August 18, 2010. https://www.clinicaleducation.org/resources/reviews/vitamin-a-friend-or-foe/.

Axe, J. "7 Bromelain Benefits, Uses & Best Food Sources." Dr. Axe. No date. https://draxe.com/6-unbelievable-health-benefits-bromelain/.

Cytowic, R. E. "The Pit in Your Stomach Is Actually Your Second Brain." *Psychology Today* [blog], January 17, 2017. https://www.psychologytoday.com/blog/the-fallible-mind/201701/the-pit-in-your-stomach-is-actually-your-second-brain.

Day, D. "The Impact of Pollution on the Skin." *MD Magazine*, January 2, 2018.

Dunn, R. "Scientists Discover That Antimicrobial Wipes and Soaps May Be Making You (and Society) Sick." *Scientific American* [blogs], July 5, 2011. https:// blogs.scientificamerican.com/guest-blog/scientists-discover-that-antimicrobial-wipes-and-soaps-may-be-making-you-and-society-sick/.

Hadazy, A. "Think Twice: How the Gut's 'Second Brain' Influences Mood and Well-Being." *Scientific American*, February 2, 2010. https://www.scientificamerican.com/article/gut-second-brain.

Islam, T., et al. "Comparative Studies on Phenolic Profiles, Antioxidant Capacities and Carotenoid Contents of Red Goji Berry (*Lycium barbarum*) and Black Goji Berry (*Lycium ruthenicum*)." *Chemistry Central Journal* 11 (2017): 59.

Jamshidi, N., and M. M. Cohen. "The Clinical Efficacy and Safety of Tulsi in Humans: A Systematic Review of the Literature." *Evidence-Based Complementary and Alternative Medicine (eCAM)* 2017 (2017): 9217567.

Jockers, D. "7 Reasons to Use Carminative Herbs." Dr. Jockers.com. No date. https://drjockers.com/7-reasons-to-use-carminative-herbs.

Kang, Y., et al. "Preventive Effects of Goji Berry on Dextran-Sulfate-Sodium-Induced Colitis in Mice." *Journal of Nutritional Biochemistry* 40 (February 2017): 70–76. Epub October 27, 2016.

Kanwal, J. "Why Poop Pulls Are in Trials as a Treatment for Obesity." Harvard University Graduate School of Arts and Sciences blog, August 22, 2016. http://sitn.hms.harvard.edu/flash/2016/second-brain-microbes-gut-may-affect-body-mind.

Koutsos, A., et al. "Apples and Cardiovascular Health—Is the Gut Microbiota a Core Consideration?" *Nutrients* 7, no. 6 (2015): 3959–3998.

MacKinnon, M. "The Science of Slow Deep Breathing." *Psychology Today* [blog], February 7, 2016. https://www.psychologytoday.com/us/blog/neuraptitude/201602/the-science-slow-deep-breathing.

Mullin, Gerald E. *The Gut Balance Revolution.* Emmaus, PA: Rodale, 2017.

O'Mahony, S. M., et al. "Serotonin, Tryptophan Metabolism and the Brain-Gut-Microbiome Axis." *Behavioural Brain Research* no. 277 (January 2015): 32–48.

Singletary, K. "Oregano: Overview of the Literature on Health Benefits." *Nutrition Today* 45, no. 3 (2010): 129–138.

Swamy, M. K., et al. "Antimicrobial Properties of Plant Essential Oils Against Human Pathogens and Their Mode of Action: An Updated Review." *Evidence-Based Complementary and Alternative Medicine* 2016 (2016): 3012462.

Taylor, P. W., et al. "Antimicrobial Properties of Green Tea Catechins." *Food Science and Technology Bulletin* 2 (2005): 71–81.

Zou, Y., et al. "Oregano Essential Oil Improves Intestinal Morphology and Expression of Tight Junction Proteins Associated with Modulation of Selected Intestinal Bacteria and Immune Status in a Pig Model." *BioMed Research International* 2016 (2016): 5436738.

Chapter 4

Bolling, B. W., et al. "The Phytochemical Composition and Antioxidant Actions of Tree Nuts." *Asia Pacific Journal of Clinical Nutrition* 19, no. 1 (2010): 117–123.

Harvard Heart Letter. "A New Spin for Spinach: A Scaffold for Working Heart Cells." Harvard Health Publishing, June 2017. https://www.health.harvard.edu/heart-health/a-new-spin-for-spinach-a-scaffold-for-working-heart-cells.

Hizo-Abes, P., et al. "Cardiovascular Disease After Escherichia coli O157:H7 Gastroenteritis." *Canadian Medical Association Journal* 185, no. 1 (2013): 70–77. Epub November 19, 2012.

Hudson, T. "Hibiscus, Hawthorn, and the Heart." *Natural Medicine Journal,* July 2011. https://www.naturalmedicinejournal.com/journal/2011-07/hibiscus-hawthorn-and-heart.

Karagozlu, N., et al. "Determination of Antimicrobial Effect of Mint and Basil Essential Oils on Survival of *E. coli* O157:H7 and *S. typhimurium* in Fresh-Cut Lettuce and Purslane." *Food Control* 22, no. 12 (2011): 1851–1855.

Ko, S.-H., et al. "Antioxidant Effects of Spinach (*Spinacia oleracea* L.) Supplementation in Hyperlipidemic Rats." *Preventive Nutrition and Food Science* 19, no. 1 (2014): 19–26.

Lovejoy, J. C., et al; "Effect of Diets Enriched in Almonds on Insulin Action and Serum Lipids in Adults with Normal Glucose Tolerance or Type 2 Diabetes." *American Journal of Clinical Nutrition* 76, no. 5 (November 1, 2002): 1000–1006.

Mercola, J. "Dry Skin Brushing: Benefits and How To." Dr. Mercola. February 24, 2014. https://articles.mercola.com/sites/articles/archive/2014/02/24/dry-skin-brushing.aspx

Moser, M. A., and O. K. Chun. "Vitamin C and Heart Health: A Review Based on Findings from Epidemiologic Studies." *International Journal of Molecular Science* 17, no. 8 (August 12, 2016): pii. http://www.mdpi.com/1422-0067/17/8/1328.

Orhan, I. E. "Phytochemical and Pharmacological Activity Profile of Crataegus oxyacantha L. (Hawthorn)—a Cardiotonic Herb." *Current Medical Chemistry* (September 18, 2016). www.ncbi.nlm.nih.gov/pubmed/27655074.

Pollock, R. L. "The Effect of Green Leafy and Cruciferous Vegetable Intake on the Incidence of Cardiovascular Disease: A Meta-analysis." *JRSM Cardiovascular Disease* 5 (2016): 2048004016661435.

Serafino, A., et al. "Stimulatory Effect of *Eucalyptus* Essential Oil on Innate Cell-Mediated Immune Response." *BMC Immunology* 9 (2008): 17.

Shmerling, R. "Your Brain on Chocolate." *Harvard Health Blog* (August 16, 2017). https://www.health.harvard.edu/blog/your-brain-on-chocolate-2017081612179

Taylor, P. W., et al. "Antimicrobial Properties of Green Tea Catechins." *Food Science and Technology Bulletin* 2 (2005): 71–81.

Wallace, T. C. "Anthocyanins in Cardiovascular Disease." *Advances in Nutrition* 2, no. 1 (January 2011): 1–7.

Yang, S. J., et al. "Effect of Eucalyptus Oil Inhalation on Pain and Inflammatory Responses after Total Knee Replacement: A Randomized Clinical Trial." *Evidence-Based Complementary and Alternative Medicine*, vol. 2013 (2013), article ID 502727. https://www.hindawi.com/journals/ecam/2013/502727/.

Chapter 5

Aucouturier, J. J., et al. "Covert Digital Manipulation of Vocal Emotion Alter Speakers' Emotional States in a Congruent Direction." *Science and Technology of Music and Sound* (January 26, 2016). http://www.pnas.org/content/pnas/early/2016/01/05/1506552113.full.pdf.

Gupta, R. "Curbside Consult: How Does the Thyroid Affect the Voice?" Osborne Head and Neck Institute. http://www.ohniww.org/how-does-the-thyroid-affect-the-voice/.

Hakanen, M., et al. "Clinical and Subclinical Autoimmune Thyroid Disease in Adult Celiac Disease." *Digestive Diseases and Sciences* 46, no. 12 (December 2001): 2631–2635. https://www.ncbi.nlm.nih.gov/pubmed/11768252.

Harris, C. "Thyroid Disease and Diet." *Today's Dietitian* 14, no. 7. http://www.todaysdietitian.com/pdf/courses/HarrisThyroidDiet.pdf.

Huang, M. J., and Y. F. Liaw. "Clinical Associations Between Thyroid and Liver Diseases." *Journal of Gastroenterology and Hepatology* 10, no. 3 (May 1995): 344–350. https://www.ncbi.nlm.nih.gov/pubmed/7548816.

Myers, A. "The Toxin, Heavy Metal, and Thyroid Connection." Amy Myers, MD, July 2015. https://www.amymyersmd.com/2015/07/the-toxin-heavy-metal-and-thyroid-connection.

Omura, Y., and S. L. Beckman. "Role of Mercury (Hg) in Resistant Infections & Effective Treatment of Chlamydia trachomatis and Herpes Family Viral Infections (and Potential Treatment for cancer) by Removing Localized Hg Deposits with Chinese Parsley and Delivering Effective Antibiotics Using Various Drug Uptake Enhancement Methods." *Acupuncture and Electrotherapeutic Research* 20, no. 3–4 (August 1995): 195–299.

"Selenium." Office of Dietary Supplements, March 2, 2018. https://ods.od.nih.gov/factsheets/Selenium-HealthProfessional.

Sharma, A. K., et al. "Efficacy and Safety of Ashwagandha Root Extract in Subclinical Hypothyroid Patients: A Double-Blind, Randomized Placebo-Controlled Trial." *Journal of Alternative and Complementary Medicine* 24, no. 3 (March 2018): 243–248.

Sharma, V., et al. "Prophylactic Efficacy of Coriandrum sativum (Coriander) on Testis of Lead-Exposed Mice." *Biological Trace Element Research* 136, no. 3 (September 2010): 337–354.

Thompson, R., et al. "Dietary Prebiotics and Bioactive Milk Fractions Improve NREM Sleep, Enhance REM Sleep Rebound and Attenuate the Stress-Induced Decrease in Diurnal Temperature and Gut Microbial Alpha Diversity." *Frontiers in Behavioral Neuroscience* (2017): 10.

Wentz, I. "Hypersomnia and Hashimoto's." Thyroid Pharmacist, August 7, 2016. https://thyroidpharmacist.com/articles/hypersomnia-and-hashimotos.

Wong, K. "The Benefits of Talking to Yourself." *New York Times*, June 8, 2017. https://www.nytimes.com/2017/06/08/smarter-living/benefits-of-talking-to-yourself-self-talk.html.

Chapter 6

"BDNF gene." Genetics Home Reference, June 5, 2018. https://ghr.nlm.nih.gov/gene/BDNF.

"Blueberries Good for Your Blood Pressure and Brain." Tufts University Nutrition Letter, April 2015. https://www.nutritionletter.tufts.edu/issues/10_16/current-articles/Blueberries-Good-for-Your-Blood-Pressure-and-Brain_1690-1.html.

Carlsen, M. H., et al. "The Total Antioxidant Content of More Than 3100 Foods, Beverages, Spices, Herbs, and Supplements Used Worldwide." *Nutrition Journal* 9 (January 22, 2010): 3.

Cavaye, J. "Does Therapeutic Massage Support Mental Well-Being?" *Medical Sociology Online* 6, no. 2 (2012): 43–50. http://www.medicalsociologyonline.org/resources/Vol6Iss2/MSo_600x_Theraputic_Massage_Cavaye.pdf.

Hugel, H. M., et al. "The Effects of Coffee Consumption on Cognition and Dementia Diseases." *Journal of Gerontology and Geriatric Research* 4 (2015): 233.

Lippi, D. "Chocolate in History: Food, Medicine, Medi-Food." *Nutrients* 5, no. 5 (2013): 1573–1584.

Lopresti, A. L. "Salvia (Sage): A Review of Its Potential Cognitive-Enhancing and Protective Effects." *Drugs in R&D* 17, no. 1 (2017): 53–64.

"Magnesium Lowers Blood Pressure, Study Suggests." ScienceDaily, March 13, 2012. https://www.sciencedaily.com/releases/2012/03/120313230354.htm.

Maione, F., et al. "In Vivo and in Vitro Biological Evaluation of the Anti-inflammatory and Analgesic Response of Carnosol and Carnosic Acid and in Silico Analysis of Their Target Interactions." *British Journal of Pharmacology*. Epub July 28, 2016.

Miller, M., and B. Shukitt-Hale. "Berry Fruit Enhances Beneficial Signaling in the Brain." *Journal of Agricultural and Food Chemistry* 60, no. 23 (2012): 5709–5715.

Moinuddin, G., et al. "Evaluation of the Anti-depressant Activity of *Myristica fragrans* (Nutmeg) in Male Rats." *Avicenna Journal of Phytomedicine* 2, no. 2 (2012): 72–78.

"Myristicin." PubChem Open Chemistry Database. https://pubchem.ncbi.nlm.nih.gov/compound/Myristicin.

Naidoo, U. "Spice Up Your Holidays with Brain-Healthy Seasonings." *Harvard Health Blog*. December 7, 2016. https://www.health.harvard.edu/blog/spice-up-your-holidays-with-brain-healthy-seasonings-2016120710734.

Rhodes, J. "Why Do I Think Better After I Exercise?" *Scientific American*. https://www.scientificamerican.com/article/why-do-you-think-better-after-walk-exercise.

Richard, D., et al. "Polyunsaturated Fatty Acids as Antioxidants." *Pharmacological Research* 57, no. 6 (June 2008): 451–455.

"Sage Improves Memory, Study Shows." ScienceDaily, September 1, 2003. https://www.sciencedaily.com/releases/2003/09/030901091846.htm.

Shukitt-Hale, B., et al. "Coffee, but Not Caffeine, Has Positive Effects on Cognition and Psychomotor Behavior in Aging." *Age* 35, no. 6 (2013): 2183–2192.

Thompson, H. "Healers Once Prescribed Chocolate Like Aspirin." *Smithsonian Magazine*, February 12, 2015. https://www.smithsonianmag.com/science-nature/healers-once-prescribed-chocolate-aspirin-180954189.

Tulleken, C. "What Does Rosemary Do to Your Brain?" *BBC News Magazine*, July 15, 2015. https://www.bbc.com/news/magazine-33519453.

Williams, R. "Iron Builds a Better Brain." *Scientist Magazine*, January 9, 2012. https://www.the-scientist.com/?articles.view/articleNo/31585/title/Iron-Builds-a-Better-Brain.

Chapter 7

Altun, I., and E. B. Kurutas. "Vitamin B Complex and Vitamin B_{12} Levels After Peripheral Nerve Injury." *Neural Regeneration Research* 11, no. 5 (2016): 842–845.

Clark, R., and S. H. Lee. "Anticancer Properties of Capsaicin Against Human Cancer." *Anticancer Research* 36, no. 3 (March 2016): 837–843.

Eteraf-Oskouei, T., and M. Najafi. "Traditional and Modern Uses of Natural Honey in Human Diseases: A Review." *Iranian Journal of Basic Medical Sciences* 16, no. 6 (2013): 731–742.

Frank, M. B., et al. "Frankincense Oil Derived from *Boswellia carteri* Induces Tumor Cell Specific Cytotoxicity." *BMC Complementary and Alternative Medicine* 9 (2009): 6.

Gregoire, C. "This Is What Sugar Does to Your Brain." *Huffington Post*, April 6, 2015. https://www.huffingtonpost.com/2015/04/06/sugar-brain-mental-health_n_6904778.html.

Hermann, N. "What Is the Function of the Various Brainwaves?" *Scientific American*, December 22, 1997. https://www.scientificamerican.com/article/what-is-the-function-of-t-1997-12-22.

Jarret, D. B., et al. "A Reexamination of the Relationship Between Growth Hormone Secretion and Slow Wave Sleep Using Delta Wave Analysis." *Biological Psychiatry* 27, no. 5 (March 1, 1990): 497–509.

Kent, S. T., et al. "Effect of Sunlight Exposure on Cognitive Function Among Depressed and Non-depressed Participants: A REGARDS Cross-sectional Study." *Environmental Health* 8 (2009): 34.

Koulivand, P. H., et al. "Lavender and the Nervous System." *Evidence-Based Complementary and Alternative Medicine (eCAM)* 2013 (2013): 681304.

Langley, W. F., and D. Mann. "Central Nervous System Magnesium Deficiency." *Archives of Internal Medicine* 151, no. 3 (March 1991): 593–596. https://www.ncbi.nlm.nih.gov/pubmed/2001142.

Lee, K.-H., et al. "Recent Progress of Research on Medicinal Mushrooms, Foods, and Other Herbal Products Used in Traditional Chinese Medicine." *Journal of Traditional and Complementary Medicine* 2, no. 2 (2012): 84–95.

Lull, C., et al. "Antiinflammatory and Immunomodulating Properties of Fungal Metabolites." *Mediators of Inflammation* 2005, no. 2 (2005): 63–80.

Mercola, J. "Magnesium: An Invisible Deficiency That Could Be Harming Your Health." Dr. Mercola, January 19, 2015. https://articles.mercola.com/sites/articles/archive/2015/01/19/magnesium-deficiency.aspx.

Muhammad, A., et al. "Neuroprotective and Anti-Aging Potentials of Essential Oils from Aromatic and Medicinal Plants." *Frontiers of Aging Neuroscience* (May 30, 2017). https://www.frontiersin.org/articles/10.3389/fnagi.2017.00168.

Qiang, Z., et al. "*Echinacea Sanguinea* and *Echinacea Pallida* Extracts Stimulate Glucoronidation and Basolateral Transfer of Bauer Alkamines 8 and 10 and Ketone 24 and Inhibit P-Glycoprotein Transporter in Caco-2 Cell." *Planta medica* 79, no. 0 (2013): 266–274.

Scholey, A., et al. "Anti-stress Effects of Lemon Balm-Containing Foods." *Nutrients* 6, no. 11 (2014): 4805–4821.

Sharma, C., et al. "Curcumin Attenuates Neurotoxicity Induced by Fluoride: An *in Vivo* Evidence." *Pharmacognosy Magazine* 10, no. 37 (2014): 61–65.

Villines, Z. "What Is the Pineal Gland?" *Medical News Today*, November 1, 2017. https://www.medicalnewstoday.com/articles/319882.php.

More on Meditation

Salleh, M. R. "Life Event, Stress and Illness." *Malaysian Journal of Medical Sciences (MJMS)* 15, no. 4 (2008): 9–18.

Schulte, B. "Harvard Neuroscientist: Meditation Not Only Reduces Stress, Here's How It Changes Your Brain." *Washington Post*, May 26, 2015. https://www.washingtonpost.com/news/inspired-life/wp/2015/05/26/harvard-neuroscientist-meditation-not-only-reduces-stress-it-literally-changes-your-brain.

ACKNOWLEDGMENTS

I am grateful for all the support and wisdom transferred to me by countless teachers from the self-help world along with the very valuable help from the small circle of modern alchemists and amazing doctors and functional medicine practitioners I've been fortunate to encounter. I would like to personally thank my alchemy teachers, including a true living alchemy master, Dennis Willian Hauck, along with many other alchemists who helped shape the thinking behind this book, including Benjamin Turale, director of the International Alchemy Guild; John Hernandez, my teacher and a longtime charter member of the Alchemy Guild; and Avery Hopkins of Kymia Arts; as well as Stephanie Wang, formerly from the Alchemist's Kitchen and Evolver.

I'm indebted to the Functional Medicine Community for their healing wisdom and helping me on my own healing journey including Sachin Patel, Tom O'Bryan, Kelly Brogan, Jared Seigler, Maya Shetreat, and many more. A big thank-you to Claire Shultz, my editor, for working her magic on the manuscript. I would also like to thank the amazing team that brought this book to life, including Andreana Bitsis, a very talented photographer; Eidia Moni, who costyled the images with me; and Cory Monji and Marguerite Imbert, who assisted us during the styling process. And as always a huge thanks always to my literary agent, Joy Tutela, who has been open to *all* of my crazy ideas that go from literary aspirations into book form, like the one you see here.

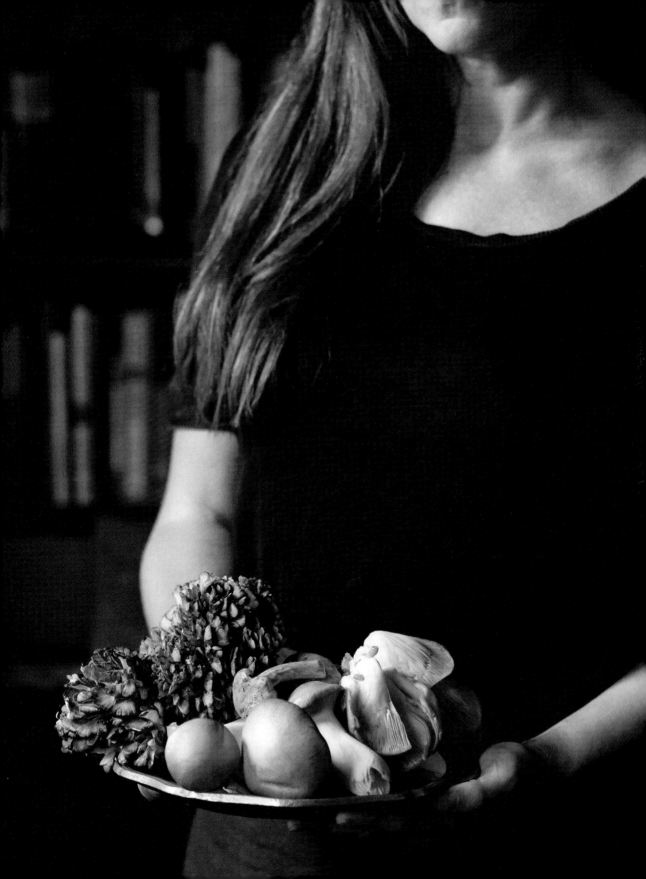

INDEX

257

263